## ABOUT DR. LYCKA'S FIRST BOOK

### *SHAPING A NEW IMAGE*

" ...the rare combination of a careful scientific and experienced medical practitioner who combines patient care with sound practical business considerations."

*David Apfelberg,* Director,
Atherton Plastic Surgery Center,
Assistant Clinical Professor of Plastic Surgery,
Stanford University

"This book is full of information you cannot find anywhere else. I think many readers will find it very useful."

*Julius Newman*, Past President,
North American Academy of
Cosmetic and Reconstructive Surgery

"Congratulations on a needed and well-written text. Your style is fun. The book is very readable and chock full of helpful, practical and important tips."

*Mark V. Dahl*
Professor and Chairman of Dermatology,
University of Minnesota Medical School

# *Skin* WORKS

## How to Restore and Keep Your Natural Beauty

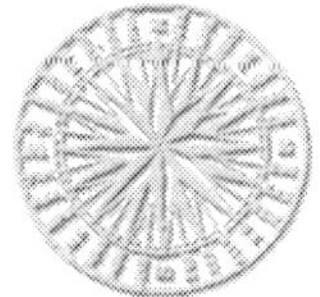

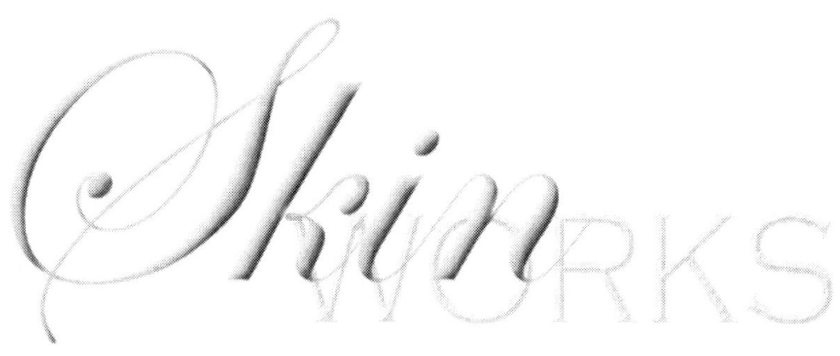

# Skin Works

How to Restore and Keep Your Natural Beauty

BARRY LYCKA M.D.

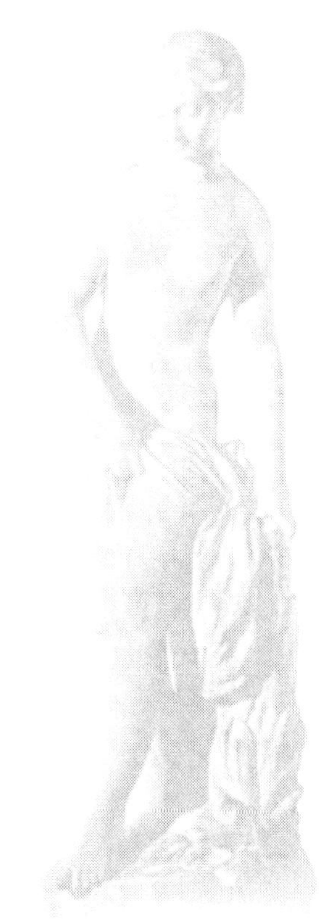

encompass
EDITIONS

**Library and Archives Canada Cataloguing in Publication**

**Lycka, Barry A. S. (Barry Allen Steven), 1956-**
**SkinWorks: How to Restore and Keep Your Natural Beauty / Barry Lycka.**

**Published 2011 by Encompass Editions, Kingston, Ontario, Canada**
**www.encompass editions.com**

**This is the first Encompass edition of the book previously published as RESTORING YOUth by CJSM Publishing Ltd, Edmonton.**

**ISBN 978-0-9865203-8-9**

**1. Skin—Care and hygiene. 2. Face—Care and hygiene. 3. Hair—Care and hygiene. 4. Beauty, Personal. 5. Surgery, Plastic. I. Title.**

**RL87.L94 2009 646.7'26 C2009-903393-3**

Printed and bound in the U.S.A.

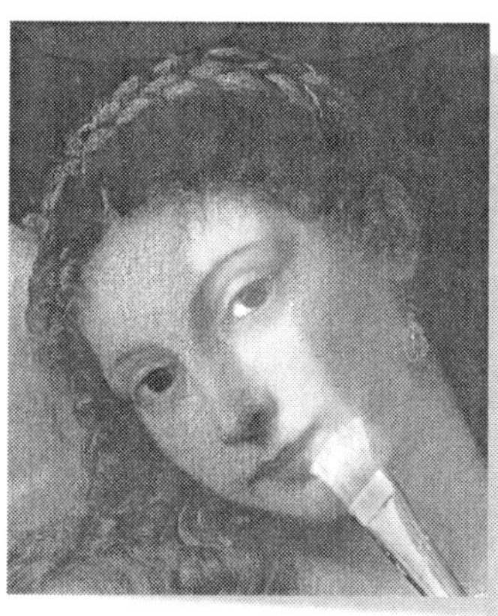

## Introduction to the Fourth Edition

I wrote the first edition of this book in 2005 and it was published in 2006 as *RESTORINGYOUth*. Since then we've gone though three editions and thousands of copies. At the time, I couldn't envisage the response it would receive.

This fourth edition, published by Encompass Editions, is entitled *SkinWorks* because I want to emphasize how central your skin is to your youthfulness and beauty. I discuss hair and breasts and liposuction, certainly, but your skin is what holds you together and it's what holds this book together. Most of us harbour a few dreams about changing ourselves for the better and I hope this book will help you achieve your dreams. Growing old should not be something we dread, but we don't have to let its have its way every day either. There is now so much new understanding of health and nutrition—and so many marvelous techniques and procedures—it's never been easier to look better and feel better.

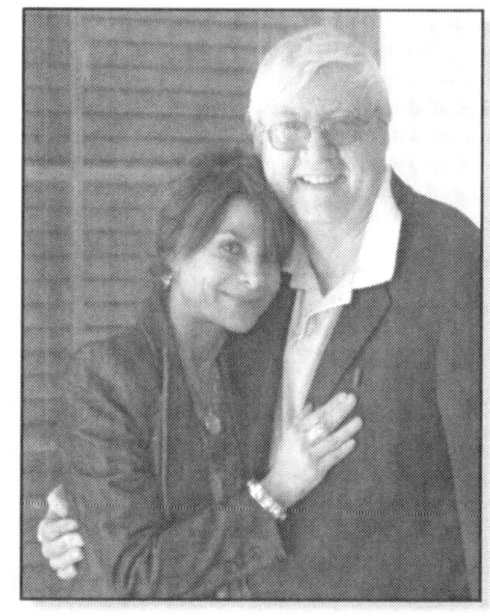

I get to know many special people in the course of my work and sometimes I learn more from them than they learn from me. A few months ago Paula Abdul shared a scary thought with me. She said, "Every woman is terrified by two things: standing in front of a microphone facing an audience and standing in front of a mirror facing herself *naked.*"

As a cosmetic dermatologist, I confront this fear daily. My job is to help people transform their looks into the looks they like. I say "help" because it's not something I can do alone; it's something my patients and I work on together. That's why I've entitled this edition *SkinWorks*.

It's very gratifying, this work. If you ask me, I'm an extremely lucky man.

*Dr. Barry Lycka*
Edmonton, January 2011

## About the Author

Barry A. S. Lycka is a cosmetic dermatologist who practices in Edmonton, Alberta, Canada, where he has lived and worked since 1979. As a young man, Dr. Lycka had almost completed a Bachelor of Arts degree at the University of Calgary when he decided to enter psychology studies. He graduated with honors in psychology, then entered medicine at the University of Alberta, graduating in 1983. He interned at the Misericordia Hospital and completed two years of internal medicine at the University of Alberta. He was chosen from hundreds of applicants to complete a fellowship in dermatology at the University of Minnesota in Minneapolis, Minnesota. He completed his residency there in 1989.

During his residency, Dr. Lycka studied laser surgery, cosmetic surgery, and Mohs micrographic surgery, an advanced technique for the removal of skin cancers. As a recognized authority in Canada and internationally, he has since completed thousands of cases in each area.

Dr. Lycka is also a recognized cosmetic-surgery authority in Canada and internationally, and a leader in offering new techniques to his clients. He was one of the first physicians to offer laser hair removal to Canada and the first in Edmonton. When refinements in laser hair removal came about, he was among the first to implement those. He developed a special interest in liposuction and received instruction on the technique from many of the world's authorities, including Patrick Lillis, Bill Hanke, William Coleman and Jeffrey Klein. He was among the first in North America to use the tumescent and extrinsic tumescent ultrasonic (XTUL) techniques, and is an acknowledged leader in the field. He was one of the first physicians to incorporate mesotherapy techniques and pioneered the use of the UltraPulse laser for resurfacing. He was also one of the first physicians in North America to offer the revolutionary thread technique of facial rejuvenation, having studied the technique in Mexico with Dr. Carl Bazan of Aguascalientes, an international expert in the technique. Dr. Lycka was one of the first surgeons in Canada to offer the advanced technique of cancer removal known as Mohs Micrographic Surgery. Recently, he has incorporated fractional resurfacing and the use of "smart lasers" in his practice.

Dr. Lycka belongs to over twenty professional societies including the prestigious Professors of Dermatological Surgery of the American Academy of Dermatology, the American Academy of Dermatology, the Canadian Dermatology Association and is vice-president of the American Society of Cosmetic Dermatology and Aesthetic Surgery. He lectures regularly and shares his expertise with international medical organizations. He also chairs a mastermind group where doctors come from all over North America to learn from his expertise. Doctor Lycka has also been a best selling author having written *Shaping A New Image: The Practice of Cosmetic Surgery*. This book has sold to thousands of doctors in over 30 different countries.

He places patient safety above all other considerations, operates an approved "non-hospital surgical facility" at First Edmonton Place in Edmonton, and maintains competency in ACLS.

In 2002, 2003, 2004 , 2005 , 2006 and 2007 Dr. Lycka has won the prestigious Consumers Choice Award for Excellence in cosmetic surgery. In 2005, Dr. Lycka founded the Canadian Skin Cancer Foundation, a nonprofit organization for the education and prevention of skin cancer. In 2006, he founded the Ethical Cosmetic Surgery Association.

Dr. Lycka is happily married to Lucie Bernier-Lycka, a family physician. They have four daughters.

# Table of Contents

# Chapter 1

# Introduction

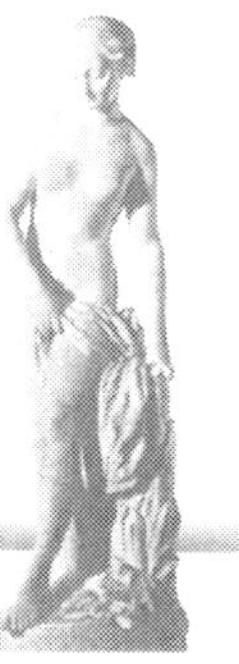

You are likely to have cosmetic surgery in your future. This is no insult or some psychic's forecast of health difficulties. On the contrary, it's a prediction based on the fact that you, like so many other perfectly healthy people, want to look and feel your best. It's based on the fact that the world of cosmetic surgery is opening to everyone and on the fact that cosmetic surgery is now easier than ever before.

Every year cosmetic surgery and related procedures grow in popularity and affordability. They are becoming less and less the luxuries of the privileged, the rich, the famous, Hollywood stars and wealthy CEOs, and more and more part of the 21st-century mainstream. Despite a flagging economy, a survey of doctors by the American Society for Aesthetic Plastic Surgery (ASAPS) shows that, in 2008, seven to 10.2 million cosmetic surgical and nonsurgical procedures were performed in the United States, representing an increase of 162 per cent over 1997, when the Society began keeping statistics. In 2008, Americans spent a total of $10 billion on plastic surgeries and $5 billion on non-surgical cosmetic procedures. Overall, the new numbers show an explosive trend. The most popular plastic surgeries were:

- Breast augmentation
- Liposuction
- Eyelid surgery
- Nose jobs
- Abdominoplasty (tummy tuck)

The most popular non-surgical procedures were:

- Botox injections

♦ Laser Hair Removal

♦ Fillers such as Hyaluronic Acid (including Hylaform, Juvederm, Perlane/Restylane)

♦ Chemical peels.

♦ Laser Skin Resurfacing

New cosmetic procedures include belly-button enhancement and breast nipple enlargement. In 2008, Women had 92% of all cosmetic procedures, while people age 35 to 50 had the most procedures (45%). People 65 and older had only 56% of all cosmetic procedures and Caucasians had 80% of all cosmetic procedures.

How widespread is all of this concern about personal appearance?

A worldwide Gallup survey, commissioned by Allergan, makers of Botox and Juvederm, included more than 5,000 adults in five countries and examined both the motivating forces and the barriers to improving facial appearance through various treatments and procedures.

"People feel quite positive, good about themselves," says Nancy Etcoff, Ph.D., social psychologist at Harvard Medical School and author of *Survival of the Prettiest*. "When they consider facial treatments, it's only small positive changes they want to make."

Etcoff reminds us that body image and a sense of one's own attractiveness are part of one's self esteem. But surprisingly, high self-esteem may actually motivate people to undergo cosmetic procedures. "People higher in self esteem are more likely to use appearance-enhancing procedures. There's not the negative motivation that one always assumes." In fact, people with low self-esteem should really see a psychotherapist to understand why they might feel this way, she adds. "They shouldn't go immediately to appearance-enhancing procedures."

Among the Gallup findings: Around the world, most people like their looks. Australia tops the list with 95% of Australians approving of their image, followed by 88% of the French, 87% of Canadians, and 85% of Americans. And if Etcoff is right, that means more and

more of us will be looking to enhance our appearance.

Some people put all this fuss down to narcissism. Others mutter something about surface appearances. But beyond such obvious—and utterly human—motives, I believe that the increase in surgical procedures speaks to people's strong desire to make positive changes in their lives, even in the face of uncertain economies and global tensions

In this book, I'll cover a myriad of procedures and treatments. I'm going to talk about your needs and wishes, literally from head to toe, and I'm confident you'll find something here to guide you toward whatever treatment you're interested in. I intend to arm you with the information and education that will lead to a happier—and even a healthier—you.

# Chapter 2

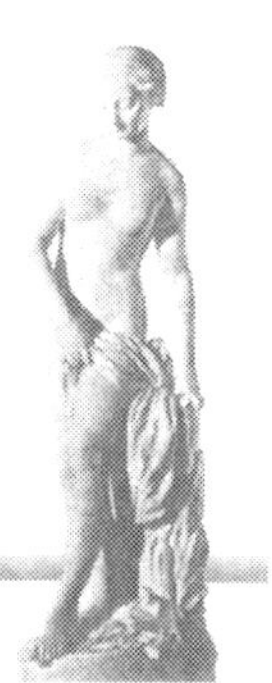

# Aging and Your Skin An Overview

## Meet Your Skin

Your skin is the largest organ of your body, made up of a complex fabric of cells, water, proteins, lipids, minerals and chemicals. Your skin weighs, on average, about six pounds, and its critical work is to protect you from infections and germs. Throughout your life, it will change constantly for better or worse, and regenerate itself approximately every 27 days.

We now know that proper care of the skin is essential if we are to maintain its health and vitality. It's easy to forget to drink that glass of water or to cleanse yourself at night when you're already tired. However, over time, those bad habits can take a toll on your skin. Each day, provide your skin with:

♦ Plenty of water.

♦ Thorough cleansing. You should perform this twice daily. At night, make sure you remove all your make-up and cleanse properly before going to bed.

♦ Balanced nutrition.

♦ Toning. After you cleanse with your bar soap or other cleanser, use a formulated toner or astringent to remove fine traces of oil, dirt and make-up that you may have missed.

♦ Moisturizing. This is necessary even for those who have oily skin. There are plenty of moisturizers on the market that are oil-free.

Over the course of your life, you must pay attention to all parts of your skin, familiarizing yourself with it and taking note of any changes that might occur, such as new moles or pigmented patches that might indicate skin cancer. Whenever you have a question or concern, see your doctor. And if you're still concerned, see a dermatologist. Your dermatologist has the specialized knowledge to help your skin.

Medical terms for various parts of your skin are commonly used today to sell skin-care products and procedures. Here's a rough guide to what those terms mean.

The *epidermis* is the thinnest layer in your skin, but it's responsible for protecting you from a potentially harsh environment. The epidermis has five layers of its own: *stratum germinativum, stratum spinosum, stratum granulosum, stratum lucidum,* and *stratum corneum*. The epidermis also hosts a variety of cell types: *keratinocytes, melanocytes* and *Langerhans cells*. Keratinocytes produce the protein known as keratin, the main component of the epidermis. Melanocytes produce your skin pigment, known as melanin. Langerhans cells prevent foreign substances from getting into your skin.

The *dermis* is the layer below the epidermis and is responsible for our wrinkles. The dermis is a complex combination of blood vessels, hair follicles, and sebaceous (oil) glands. *Fibroblasts* are among the cells of the dermis and they synthesize *collagen* and *elastin,* two proteins necessary for skin health because they offer support and elasticity. The dermis also contains pain and touch receptors.

*Collagen* is the most abundant protein in the skin, making up 75% of all skin mass. Collagen is also your fountain of youth, responsible for warding off wrinkles and fine lines. Over time, environmental factors and aging diminish your body's ability to produce collagen.

When you hear the word *elastin*, think elastic. This protein is found with collagen in the dermis and is responsible for giving structure to your skin and organs. As with collagen, elastin is affected by time and the elements. Diminished levels of this protein cause your skin to wrinkle and sag.

Keratin is the strongest protein in your skin and it too is found in the epidermis and the dermis. It's also dominant in hair and nails. Keratin is what gives your skin its necessary rigidity.

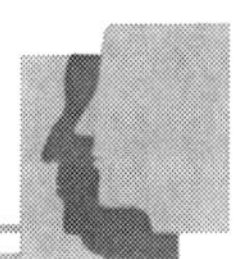

Finally, in this layer is hyaluronic acid (HA)—the "sea" that everything else floats in.

The *hypodermis,* also known as the *subcutis or hypodermis*, is the deepest layer. Reduction of tissue in the hypodermis is what causes your skin to sag. The hypodermis hosts sweat glands, fat cells and collagen cells and is responsible for conserving your body's heat and protecting your vital inner organs.

## YOUR AGING SKIN

Our skin is proof that life is about change. It's at the mercy of many forces: sun, harsh weather, and our own bad habits. However, we *can* take steps to help our skin stay supple and fresh looking.

How your skin ages will depend on a variety of factors: your lifestyle, diet, heredity, and personal habits. Are you a smoker or did you ever smoke? Smoking can produce free radicals, once-healthy oxygen molecules that are now overactive and unstable. These damage the skin and may cause cancers and premature aging. But wrinkled and spotted skin can be the result of normal aging too, and exposure to the sun (photo-aging), and loss of subcutaneous support (the fatty tissue between your skin and muscle). Other factors include stress, gravity, daily facial movement, obesity, and even sleep position.

To a cosmetic surgeon aging results in three *d*s: decay, descent and deflation.

When we speak of *decay*, we mean that the components of the body start to break down. We develop lentigos ("sun spots"), for example, loss of elasticity, the more serious lesions of skin cancers—and our body's healing ability begins to decay too.

*Descent* refers to the way everything falls as we age. Skin literally migrates, with jowls, wrinkles and facial wrinkles developing as a consequence.

*Deflation* refers to the fact that the bones in our face get smaller as we age. This results in the sunken appearance we develop around our eyes and cheeks. All of these must be addressed if we want to retain a youthful appearance.

**SKIN CHANGES WITH AGE**

♦ Skin becomes rougher.
♦ Skin develops growths such as benign and malignant tumors.
♦ Skin becomes slack. The loss of the elastic tissue (elastin and collagen) in the skin with age causes the skin to hang loosely.
♦ Skin becomes more transparent as we age. This is caused by thinning of the epidermis, the surface layer.
♦ Skin becomes more fragile as we age. This is caused by a flattening of the area where the epidermis and dermis (layer of skin under the epidermis) come together—the dermal-epidermal junction.
♦ Skin becomes more easily bruised due to the thinning of blood vessel walls.

Over time, the sun's ultraviolet (UV) light damages the elastin fibers in the skin. The breakdown of elastin fibers causes the skin to sag, stretch, and lose its ability to snap back after stretching. The skin also bruises and tears more easily and takes longer to heal. Sun damage may not show when you're young, but it will later in life.

Nothing can completely undo sun damage, but the skin *can* repair itself to a certain extent and you *can* protect yourself from sun exposure and skin cancer, and begin "turning back" the clock on your aging skin. You can effectively delay changes associated with aging by protecting yourself from the sun and by treating your skin properly.

Currently, doctors recommend sun blocks with an SPF of at least 15. I personally prefer sunscreens with an SPF of 30 to 60. Sun damage is so widespread in our population, I predict that, within the next few years, sun block will most likely become part of all North American women's daily cosmetic routine; women will put it on as regularly as they do a daily moisturizer. Men will eventually do the same. If they don't, they'll pay the piper, with aging and sagging skin

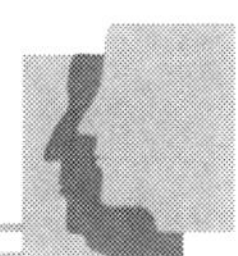

or worse. As the old television commercials said: You can pay me now or you can pay me later. It's your choice.

We'll come back to the sun in the next section. But let's look further at that long list of the skin's enemies.

With aging, loss of fat below the skin in the cheeks, temples, chin, nose and eye area may result in loosening skin, sunken eyes and a "skeletal" appearance. Bone loss, mostly around the mouth and chin, may become evident after age 60 and cause puckering of the skin around the mouth. Cartilage loss in the nose causes drooping of the nasal tip and accentuation of the bony structures in the nose.

Gravity, facial movement and sleep position are the secondary factors that contribute to changes in the skin. When the skin loses its elasticity, gravity causes drooping of the eyebrows and eyelids, looseness and fullness under the cheeks and jaw (jowls and "double chin"), and longer ear lobes.

Facial movement lines become more visible after the skin starts losing its elasticity, usually as people reach their 30s and 40s. Lines may appear horizontally on the forehead, vertically on the skin above the root of the nose (glabellas), or as small curved lines on the temples, upper cheeks and around the mouth.

Sleep creases result from the way the head is positioned on the pillow and may become more visible after the skin starts losing its elasticity. Sleep creases are commonly located on the side of the forehead, starting above the eyebrows to the hairline near the temples, as well as on the middle of the cheeks. Changing sleep position may improve these sleep creases or prevent them from becoming worse.

Smokers tend to have more wrinkles than nonsmokers of the same age, complexion, and history of sun exposure. The reason for this difference is unclear, although it may be because smoking interferes with normal blood flow in the skin or because smoking causes free radical formation.

Dry skin and itching is common in later life. About 85% of older people develop "winter itch" due to dry, heated indoor air. The loss of sweat and oil glands as we age may also worsen dry skin. Anything that further dries the skin—the overuse of soaps, antiperspirants, perfumes, or hot baths—will make the problem worse. If your skin is very dry and itchy, you should see a doctor because this condition can affect your sleep, cause irritability, or even be a symptom of a disease. For example, diabetes and kidney disease can cause itching. Some medicines make the itchiness worse.

Skin changes in other ways. In women, as estrogen decreases, skin tends to lose its elasticity and becomes thinner because it is no longer able to retain as much water. Sweat and oil glands also produce less moisture, which is what causes the skin to gradually dry, wrinkle, and sag.

Good moisturizers and skin care will certainly help to keep your skin more elastic. But the number one factor that damages the skin and speeds up your skin's natural aging process is the sun. If you cut down your sun exposure, you can dramatically reduce visible aging of your skin. Period. The bad news is that much of the sun's damage on your skin is cumulative damage from many years of exposure. In fact, many researchers believe that when it comes to visible signs of aging, estrogen loss is only a small factor. Sun exposure may be a far more important factor because ultraviolet rays break down collagen and elastin fibers in the skin, causing it to sag. This is also what puts you at risk for skin cancer, the most notorious of which is melanoma, one of the most aggressive and malignant of all cancers.

Other sun-related problems traditionally linked to estrogen loss include "liver spots," light brown or tan splotches that develop on the face, neck, and hands as you age. These spots have nothing to do with the liver; they are "sun spots" caused by sun exposure. They are sometimes the result of hormone replacement therapy (HRT), in which case they are called hyperpigmentation.

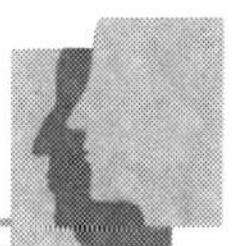

## SLOWING THE AGING PROCESS

We are no longer willing to sit passively and let time have its way with us. We want to slow time and limit its ravages.

### Take Action Now

You can fight aging right now through lifestyle changes that anyone can manage. Scientists tell us that advances in medicine and public health are enabling people to live longer and stay in good shape. It's not uncommon these days to find men and women in their 90s enjoying a 30-minute walk or playing golf. The Center for Disease Control and Prevention recently reported that people are now living an average of 30 years longer than they did in 1900. Increasing human life expectancy may no longer be a fantasy.

But for scientists, helping people live more healthfully, not necessarily longer, is the more realistic goal. You can't prevent the aging process itself. But you can slow it down. In one study, thousands of people across the world are helping researchers discover the keys to healthy aging. Every year or two the study participants, ranging in age from 18 to 90 years, complete a battery of tests that measure everything from how well their brains function to how fast their hearts beat. Not surprisingly, these scientists are finding that a key to healthy aging is lifestyle. Smokers, couch potatoes and people who subsist on fast food will age faster and fall ill sooner.

Recently, the documentary movie *Super Size Me* provided a graphic illustration of this fact. In *Super Size Me*, the filmmaker eats all meals at McDonalds every day for 30 days. He becomes obese, depressed and develops blood pressure problems. At the end of the experiment, his physician advises him that his liver resembles that of an alcoholic. It takes him another 14 months to lose the weight and recover his health.

**Eat Less**

According to the caloric-restriction theory, another key to youth may simply be eating less. This theory, which holds that people can live longer if they cut back on the number of calories they consume each day, gained popularity when researchers showed that mice that eat less can increase their maximum lifespan from 39 months (the equivalent of 110 human years, the maximum human lifespan) to 56 months (162 human years). Researchers hope their work with mice will be applicable to humans but, since the human lifespan is so long, similar research in humans has not yet been completed. Nonetheless, the theory got a boost in 1991 when subjects entered Biosphere 2, a sealed three-acre, glass-domed space outside Tucson, Arizona. Biosphere 2 contained several ecological climates and environments, such as a rain forest and a savanna, as well as scientific laboratories. For two years the subjects lived on a diet of 1,800 calories a day that consisted of fruits, vegetables, grains, beans and some meat. They recorded significant decreases in their blood pressure and cholesterol. These and other physiological signs suggest that the aging process may be slowed by up to 50 percent.

It may be that people can benefit from cutting their caloric intake by a mere 10 percent. However, those restricting their calories must choose foods more wisely to ensure that the diets include enough nutrients, and certainly this sort of diet must be practiced with care. Pregnant women and children, for example, should not embark on calorically restricted diets. Yet in general, people who want to live longer don't have to wait for any more research and should just get started by cutting back on their calories now.

**Exercise**

This won't come as news—health-wise people combine their reduced caloric intake with exercise. Staying physically active is the best strategy for staying young, healthy and fit in the face of basic biology and the natural progression of life. The fight isn't easy. It

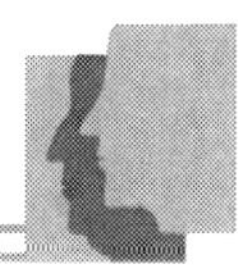

requires an unwavering discipline and motivation to exercise regularly, eat right and maintain a positive attitude, elements crucial in holding back diseases associated with our enemy—old age.

You need to go on the offensive, making exercise one of your weapons of choice. It's a sound guideline to work out three times a week, with each routine including 20 minutes on a cardiovascular machine and 40 minutes of weights and other muscle-strengthening exercises. With a trainer's help and good humor, you'll find exercise rewarding, allowing you to stay active and continue doing as much as you'd like.

Exercise is one of the most important factors in reducing the effects of the aging process. Exercise offsets the body's natural tendency to gain body fat and lose muscle and bone mass, which starts at age 35. Without exercise, loss of muscle strength and diminished cardiovascular fitness quickly follow, making any type of physical activity more difficult.

In addition to helping a person stay trim, regular exercise also reduces the risk for heart disease, osteoporosis, diabetes, obesity and depression, while improving self-confidence, sleep quality and self-esteem. For example, one famous study examined women age 50 to 70 who had always been sedentary. After one year of strength training twice a week, the women became 75 percent stronger, lost fat, and gained muscle and bone mass in their hips and spines. However, no matter how young you might feel, you should not spend more than two hours every day on cardiovascular machines, in the weight room, or playing racquetball or other sports. Even if you are eating foods that are low in fat and packed with nutrients, excessive exercise can have a detrimental effect.

Men with a waist of more than 40 inches and women with a waist of more than 35 inches are at increased risk for osteoarthritis, heart disease, cancer, diabetes and a score of other chronic diseases. However, the benefits of a healthy lifestyle go beyond avoiding chronic disease and premature death. Dedication to exercise and a healthy diet means feeling young and staying active for as long as our genes, our bodies and time itself allows.

## Your Diet: More than Skin Deep

The skin is the outer reflection of your inner health. Moist, clear, glowing skin is a sign of good diet, while dry, pale, scaly or oily skin may result when diet is not up to par. Fortunately, the eating habits that work best for staying healthy in other respects are also the next best thing to a fountain of youth for our skin.

In a study published in a 2001 *Journal of the American College of Nutrition*, researchers looked at the current diets of more than 400 adults aged 70 and older living in Australia, Greece and Sweden. The researchers found that even when they factored in age and smoking, diet still played a role in the wrinkling of sun-exposed skin. Whether they were dark-skinned or fair-skinned, whether they lived in sun-drenched Australia or sun-deprived Sweden, people who ate plenty of wholesome foods such as green leafy vegetables, beans, olive oil, nuts, and multigrain breads were less prone to wrinkling that those who consumed a lot of butter, red meat, and sugary confections.

### *Your Skin and Nutrients*

Just about every nutrient has a role in maintaining healthy skin. Vitamin C helps build collagen, the "scaffolding" between the tissues of our body. Poor intake of this vitamin can cause bruising, loss of skin strength and elasticity, and poor healing of cuts and scrapes. Just one daily glass of orange juice or a bowl of strawberries supplies all the vitamin C you need. Healthy skin also needs the B vitamins found in whole grains, milk and wheat germ, vitamins that help speed wound-healing and prevent dry, flaky or oily skin. Vitamin A in dark orange or green vegetables and fruits, egg yolks and liver, maintains epithelial tissues such as skin, thus helping to prevent premature wrinkling or bumpy, sandpaper-like skin. Vitamin D in milk may help curb symptoms of psoriasis. Zinc in meat, seafood, and legumes aids in the

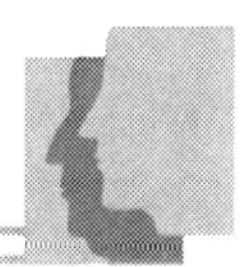

healing of cuts and scrapes. Water keeps the skin moist and regulates normal function of the oil glands. The list of nutrients that benefit the skin is almost endless.

Your skin needs a constant supply of water and oxygen, though that doesn't mean you have to take your showers in the open air. Rather, these nutrients need to be supplied through your blood, which provides other nutrients and removes waste products. It takes an ample amount of many nutrients to build and maintain healthy red blood cells and other blood factors. Those nutrients include protein, iron and copper, plus folic acid, other B vitamins, and vitamins C and E. A deficiency of any of these, especially iron, reduces the oxygen-carrying capacity of the blood, suffocating the skin and leaving it pale and drawn.

Some nutrients directly affect the health of your skin. Repairing damaged skin requires protein, zinc, and vitamins A, C, and K. Vitamin D, a vitamin actually made in the skin through the action of sunlight, has important roles in human health, including modulation of neuromuscular and immune function, reduction of inflammation, and the possible reduction of risk of certain cancers. Linoleic acid is a fat in vegetable oils that also helps restore damaged skin and keep skin smooth and moist. On the other hand, a high-fat diet may increase the risk for developing skin cancer. The solution to these seemingly contradictory findings is simple: Consume an overall low-fat diet and follow the basic guidelines I'm going to summarize below.

Consume minimally processed foods daily: fresh fruits and vegetables, whole grain breads and cereals, and cooked, dried beans and peas, with two to three servings of nonfat milk and a small amount of extra-lean meat or fish. Include several servings daily of antioxidant-rich foods such as oranges for vitamin C, dark green leafy vegetables and apricots for beta carotene, and wheat germ for vitamin E. Include one linoleic acid-rich food in your daily diet. Safflower oil, nuts, avocado and seeds are all sources. Take 1000 to 2000 I.U. of Vitamin D a day. Drink six to eight glasses of water daily. Avoid repeated bouts of weight loss and regain, since weight cycling can result in premature sagging, stretch marks, and wrinkling. Take a moderate-dose vitamin and mineral supplement.

### *Diet and Free Radicals*

Much of the so-called aging of the skin is really a result of long-term exposure to sun, tobacco smoke, and ozone. Environmental pollutants generate the highly damaging oxygen fragments called free radicals that we discussed earlier. These erode skin much as water rusts metal. Free radicals also damage collagen, the protein latticework that maintains the skin's firmness and suppleness. The result is a condition called photo-aging, which includes dryness, loss of elasticity, and the appearance of fine lines and wrinkles.

Free radicals generated by sun exposure also damage the genetic structure of skin cells and so contribute to the development of cancer. Antioxidant nutrients, including vitamins C and E and beta carotene, show promise in slowing the rate of free-radical damage to the skin. People who daily consume five or more antioxidant-rich foods—spinach, for instance, and sweet potatoes, tomatoes, cantaloupe, grapefruit, and carrots—stockpile these health-enhancing nutrients in their tissues and develop fewer skin cancers. Of course, the antioxidants are effective only if you combine this healthful diet with other risk-control habits such as avoiding sun and using sunscreen lotions.

### *Diet and Aging*

But diet also plays an integral role in preventing old-age diseases. There are several key nutrients important in maintaining health that older people should take care to include in their diet: calcium and vitamin D, which prevent osteoporosis; vitamin E, which studies are showing reduces the risk of heart disease and Alzheimer's disease; and vitamin $B_{12,}$ which guards against anemia and nerve dysfunction.

In general, getting recommended amounts of nutrients in the daily diet keeps the immune system healthy and helps the body defend

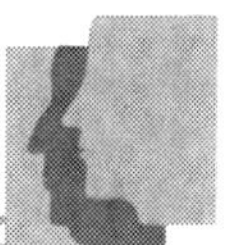

itself against infection and cancer—and premature aging.

**Stop Smoking Now**

The nicotine in cigarettes not only causes your heart's arteries to constrict, thereby increasing the risk of a heart attack, but also causes the small arterioles and capillaries in your face to constrict. As we've seen, this may be the cause of the wrinkling and premature aging often observed in smokers. The next time you're at a party, take a look at the people who are smoking. They often look much older than their age.

**Limit Your Stress**

Chronic emotional stress also causes the same constriction of your blood vessels as nicotine, so practicing stress-management techniques on a regular basis may help you look younger and feel better.

**Human Growth Hormone**

Researchers are taking great interest in the hormones that may be intimately involved in the aging process. The human growth hormone has been studied for 20 years. Young people lacking this hormone display premature signs of aging, which disappear once they take artificial growth hormone. On the other hand, previous studies have found that older men who took the hormone had an increase in muscle mass and a decrease in fat. Researchers are also studying the sex hormones—testosterone and estrogen—that decline as the growth hormone starts decreasing at about age 30. These too may play a role in the symptoms of aging. Testosterone, when given as a supplement, has been shown to slow aging in males. When, in the next few years, researchers finish analyzing the data, they expect to uncover more about whether the growth hormone—by itself or in combination with a sex hormone—can increase muscle strength and aerobic fitness and so offset health problems such as heart disease, osteoporosis and diabetes. As more is discovered, I'll report it in later editions of this book, but in the meantime, MDs recommend that people abstain from taking growth hormone supplements. Researchers need to learn more about this hormone. We already know that, in addition to the benefits that may be associated with these hormones, they may have such side effects as high blood pressure, headaches and carpal tunnel syndrome.

**Andro Strikes Out**

One popular "cure" for aging or wrinkles was recently proved to be a total fiction. The controversial supplement used by baseball slugger Mark McGwire during his 1998 record-breaking home-run streak has struck out. In eight or so studies, researchers found no positive health benefits or any evidence that androstenedione—"andro" for short—did what was claimed, namely increase muscle mass, strength, libido, sexual performance, or athletic performance.

Advocates claim is that the body uses andro to make more of the male hormone testosterone. This has not been substantiated. Many studies find androstenedione doesn't boost testosterone in men, but what it *does* do at the popular 200-milligram dose is boost *estrogen* levels and disrupt a natural hormonal balance. The result can be an increase in the risk of heart disease, prostate cancer and other health problems. One trial, funded after McGwire's record by the Major League Baseball Association and the Major League Baseball Players Association, and published recently in the *Journal of the American Medical Association*, found androstenedione raised testosterone *and* estrogen levels at the 300 milligram dose, but did not raise testosterone at lower doses. The effects moreover were fleeting and there was no evidence that andro builds muscle mass or aids in athletics.

After failing to claim credit for McGwire's mighty bat and biceps, marketers quietly repositioned androstenedione as an anti-aging supplement, selling it on Internet sites and at anti-aging clinics. Since there's a natural waning in testosterone levels as men age, the theory is boosting that these levels can offset or reverse the effects of aging.

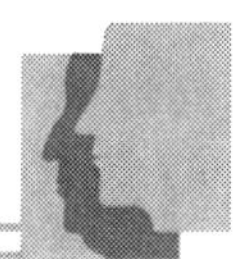

Even if androstenedione was successful at boosting testosterone, there's no evidence that it would help slow aging.

Nor is there evidence that andro does anything to favorably alter health. In the absence of a true hormonal imbalance, supplemental hormones can disrupt the hormonal profile in both men and women. Basically, the hormones you don't want to increase do increase. In men, andro does a fantastic job of raising estrogen levels. In addition, in women, it would likely boost testosterone levels. That's not what most women want.

Why is this medication still around? Androstenedione is dangerous and findings are consistent with previous research suggesting *no* benefit from androstenedione supplementation. There are two things you need to understand about andro: First, it is an anabolic steroid and the only reason that is still on the shelves today is because it was not included in the Anabolic Steroid Control Act of 1990. Andro has no known medical use, and nobody was using it at the time medications such as this were banned, so it wasn't put on the list of banned substances. Second, it just doesn't work, and that also applies to its alleged anti-aging benefits. For athletic performance, it seemingly provides all the negative aspects of other anabolic steroids but none of the positive ones.

Remember, if something sounds too good to be true, it probably is.

### *Steroids*

Professional athletes have used anabolic steroids to enhance their physical performance. They help build muscle mass but at great cost: they can alter an individual's psyche and wreak havoc on the internal organs.

Steroids have been banned by most professional groups. Ben Johnson and Florence Griffith Joyner are just two who have been caught and lost their medals as a result. the same fate has befallen stars in baseball, football, and cycling. Needless to say, you're not going to follow their foolish examples.

## Breakthroughs to Come

Research may someday help increase the human lifespan as science develops drugs that slow the aging process at the genetic level. Researchers have already developed genetically engineered muscle cells in mice that stimulate the body to produce blood vessels. Reinvigorated blood vessels may prevent the development of heart disease and poor circulation, as well as delay the muscle atrophy and slow healing that afflict older people. Scientists will begin clinical trials in the near future to see if these genetically-altered cells can increase blood-vessel development in people.

Although we now know much about the genetics of aging, actual genetic therapies are a thing of the future. Tomorrow's anti-aging therapies aren't going to happen today.

# Sun Damage and Skin Cancer

## Look Out! Here Comes the Sun!

A Beatles song urged listeners to "follow the sun" but the Beatles weren't thinking about your skin. Few people were in those days.

The most important tip I can offer to anyone who wants to avoid skin problems—including cancer—is to use sunscreen every day. A number of studies have shown that perhaps 80% of what makes a person's face look older is related to sun exposure. If you begin using sunscreen when you are young, you may look younger for a much longer time. And the incidence of melanoma, a potentially fatal skin cancer, is directly linked to sun exposure: the regular use of sunscreen may help you *live* longer as well as *look* younger. I recommend a minimum SPF of 15 to my patients, one that blocks both the long ultraviolet (UVA) rays and the even more dangerous short (UVB) rays. I prefer an SPF of 30 to 60. As the ozone layer continues to be depleted, the use of sunscreen becomes even more important.

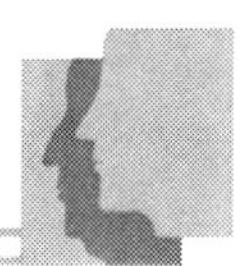

***Bad News—Indoors or Out***

It doesn't save you from tanning risks when you go to indoor tanning salons. You need to be smarter than the folks out there who are so desperate for a good tan that they'll do anything to get one. A 2002 survey of 489 students at Indiana University shows 92% of users know that tanning beds are linked to premature aging and skin cancer. But 71% said they used the beds because there wasn't enough time to tan outside, and 61% said they used them to prepare for vacations (the so-called base tan). The researchers also asked students some basic questions about skin cancer and moles, so that researchers could rate their knowledge about skin cancer detection. Most students who used tanning beds knew that skin cancer and premature aging were possible complications. More than 75% believed that tanning lamps are unsafe or were unsure of their safety.

Despite adequate knowledge of the adverse effects of UV exposure, university students freely and frequently use tanning lamps, primarily to attain a desired cosmetic appearance. And, strikingly, students in one study who had a positive family history of skin cancer were 1.5 times more likely to use tanning lamps than those *without* such a history. The dangers of tanning-lamp use seem to be widely known, yet have little bearing on behavior patterns.

If students are going to quit this risky behavior, it's going to take a fundamental change in the way society views tans. The Indiana study, which appeared in the October 2003 issue of the *Archives of Dermatology*, adds to a growing body of evidence showing that adults and adolescents, especially young women, are using tanning beds regularly, putting themselves at high risk of skin cancer.

At least *you* know better.

## Skin Cancer—No Minor Concern

Many people love the warm sun. The sun's rays make us feel good, and in the short term, make us look good. But our love affair isn't a reciprocal one: exposure to sun causes most of the wrinkles and age spots on our faces. Consider this: a woman at age 40 who has protected her skin from the sun may have the skin we expect a 30-year-old to have!

We often associate a glowing complexion with good health, but skin color obtained from being in the sun—or in a tanning booth—actually accelerates the effects of aging and increases your risk of developing skin cancer. Sun exposure causes most of the skin changes that we think of as a normal part of aging. Over time, the sun's ultraviolet (UV) light damages the fibers in the skin called elastin. When these fibers break down, the skin begins to sag, stretch, and lose its ability to go back into place after stretching. The skin also bruises and tears more easily and takes longer to heal. So while sun damage to the skin may not be apparent when you're young, it will definitely show later in life.

***Exposure to the Sun Causes:***

- Pre-cancerous (actinic keratosis) and cancerous (basal cell carcinoma, squamous cell carcinoma and melanoma) skin lesions that result from a breakdown in the skin's immune function and damage to the skin cells
- Benign tumors
- Fine and coarse wrinkles
- Freckles
- Discolored areas of the skin, called mottled pigmentation
- Sallowness—a yellow discoloration of the skin
- Telangiectasias—a dilation of small blood vessels under the skin
- Elastosis—a destruction of the elastic tissues that causes lines and wrinkles.

Skin cancer—the uncontrolled growth of abnormal skin cells—is the most prevalent form of all cancers in the U.S. and the number of cases continues to rise. There are three main types of skin cancer: basal cell carcinoma, squamous cell carcinoma and melanoma. Basal cell and squamous cell cancers are less serious types and make

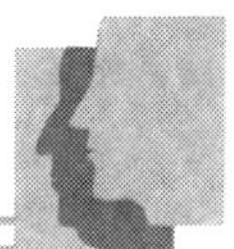

up 95% of all skin cancers. Also referred to as non-melanoma skin cancers, they are highly curable when treated early. Melanoma, made up of abnormal skin-pigment cells called melanocytes, is the most serious form of skin cancer and causes 75% of all skin cancer deaths. If not detected and treated quickly, it can spread to other organs and is difficult to control.

Ultraviolet (UV) radiation from the sun is the number-one cause of skin cancer, but UV light from tanning beds is just as harmful. Exposure to sunlight during the winter months puts you at the same risk as exposure during the summertime.

Cumulative sun exposure causes mainly basal-cell and squamous-cell skin cancer, while episodes of severe sunburns, usually before age 18, can cause melanoma later in life. Other less common causes are repeated X-ray exposure, scars from burns or disease and occupational exposure to certain chemicals.

Although anyone can get skin cancer, the risk is greatest for people who have fair or freckled skin that burns easily, light eyes and blond or red hair. Darker skinned individuals are also susceptible to all types of skin cancer, although their risk is substantially lower.

Aside from complexion, other risk factors include having a family history or personal history of skin cancer, having an outdoor job and living in a sunny climate. A history of severe sunburns and an abundance of large and irregularly-shaped moles are risk factors unique to melanoma.

The most common warning sign of skin cancer is a change on the skin, typically a new mole or skin lesion or a change in an existing mole. Basal cell carcinoma may appear as a small, smooth, pearly or waxy bump on the face ears and neck; or as a flat, pink/red- or brown-colored lesion on the trunk or arms and legs.

Squamous cell carcinoma can appear as a firm, red nodule, or as a rough, scaly flat lesion that may itch, bleed and become crusty. Both basal cell and squamous cell cancers mainly occur on areas of the skin frequently exposed to the sun, but can occur anywhere.

Melanoma usually appears as a pigmented patch or bump. It may resemble a normal mole, but usually has a more irregular appearance. When looking for melanoma, use the ABCD rule to remember the signs to watch for:

♦ Asymmetry—the shape of one half doesn't match the other
♦ Border—edges are ragged or blurred
♦ Color—uneven shades of brown, black, tan, red, white or blue
♦ Diameter—a significant change in size (greater than 6mm).

Skin cancer is diagnosed only by performing a biopsy. This involves taking a sample of the tissue, which is then placed under a microscope and examined by a dermatopathologist, a doctor who specializes in examining skin cells. Sometimes a biopsy may remove all of the cancer tissue and no further treatment is needed.

Treatment of skin cancer depends on the type and extent of the disease. Treatment is individualized and is determined by the type of skin cancer, its size and location and the patient's preference. Standard treatments for non-melanoma skin cancer (basal cell or squamous cell carcinomas) include:

♦ Mohs surgery (for high-risk non-melanoma skin cancers)—excision of cancer and some extra tissue. This has the highest cure rate. Since 1986 I have done at least 4000 cancers by this method.
♦ Electrodessication and curettage—physically scraping away the skin cancer cells followed by electrosurgery
♦ Cryosurgery or freezing
♦ Laser therapy
♦ Drugs (chemotherapy, biological response modifiers to destroy cancer cells)

Standard treatments for melanoma skin cancer include:

♦ Wide surgical excision
♦ Sentinel lymph node mapping (for deeper lesions)—to determine if the melanoma has spread to local lymph nodes
♦ Drugs (chemotherapy, biological response modifiers)
♦ Radiation therapy

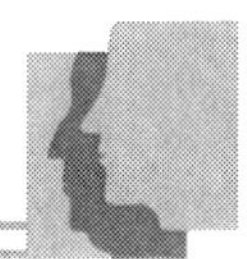

♦ New methods are sometimes used to treat skin cancer in clinical trials.

Although the skin can sometimes repair itself, nothing can completely undo sun damage. For this reason, it's never too late to begin protecting yourself from the sun. Your skin does change with age—for example, you sweat less and your skin can take longer to heal—but you can delay these changes by staying out of the sun. Follow these tips to help prevent skin cancer:

♦ Apply sunscreen with a sun protection factor (SPF) of 30 or greater 30 minutes before sun exposure and then every few hours thereafter.

♦ Select cosmetic products and contact lenses that offer UV protection.

♦ Wear sunglasses with total UV protection.

♦ Avoid direct sun exposure as much as possible during the peak UV-radiation hours between 10:00 A.M. to 3:00 P.M.

♦ Perform skin self-exams regularly to become familiar with existing growths and to notice any changes or new growths.

Studies show that currently 80% of a person's lifetime sun exposure is acquired before age 18. As a parent, be a good role model and foster skin cancer prevention habits in your child.

Yet it turns out that you're one of those who still want to look brown. Good news for you: modern science has provided a great way to do so. It's called a "fantasy tan" and it consists of having a special spray of DHEA applied to your skin in the doctor's office. Ask your dermatologist about it.

## Acne and Other Skin Ailments

### Acne

As adolescents, we would expect Mother Nature to aid us in our sudden desire to look as good as we can. But Mother Nature often conspires instead to make us look as bad as we'll look in our entire life. Our face becomes a general plague zone.

Many an adolescent has been challenged by acne and certainly it couldn't come at a worse time developmentally. Our peers become all-important. What do they think about us? Who has what status in the group? Who's up and who's down? Interest in dating is beginning to peak. Hormones are running wild and tend to make every issue more emotional and more intensely felt. It's a time of tremendous self-consciousness as teens try to figure out just who they are and who they want to be.

In that context, acne can seem like just about the worst thing that could happen to a person. And, in many cases, it can continue into adulthood. Acne vulgaris (acne) is a common skin condition that can affect people of all ages, although teenagers develop acne most often. Acne affects about 80% of people at some point in their lives, and it is reported that problems with acne are responsible for more than 30% of all visits to dermatologists.

Acne is a disorder that occurs when the sebaceous glands in a person's skin make too much oil (sebum). The oil combines with cells that line the walls of these glands and so clogs the person's skin pores. Clogging of pores leads to pimples—whiteheads or blackheads—that usually occur on the face, neck, shoulders, back, or chest. Pimples that are large and deep are called cystic lesions. Cystic lesions can cause painful infections and lead to scarring.

It is not entirely clear what causes a person's body to produce too much oil or not properly shed dead skin cells. Outbreaks of acne may be linked to hormones, genetics, or bacteria. We do know one thing for certain, however: acne is not caused by eating too much chocolate or oily foods.

Moderate to severe acne can cause embarrassment and self-esteem problems and sometimes depression. Only one-third of teenagers with acne seek treatment, although most report that acne causes them to have a poor self-image.

Acne can range from mild to severe. A person may have only

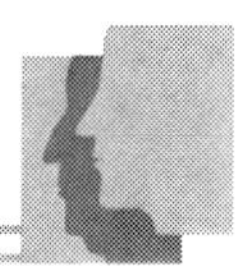

occasional bouts of pimples or they may be constant. Treatment for acne is based on the severity of the outbreak and how much it affects a person's appearance. Although there is no known cure for acne, if it is mild to moderate, home care with non-prescription products such as lotions, cleansing soaps, or washes may be enough to control the condition.

If acne is severe or has not improved after six to eight weeks of home care, treatment by a doctor may be necessary. A person may want to seek medical assistance sooner if there is a strong family history of acne or if the acne developed at an early age. If a person has mild acne but is emotionally affected by it, treatment may be needed.

The goal of treatment is to reduce or eliminate outbreaks, control the progression of inflammation and cyst formation, and prevent scarring. Home care of acne and use of non-prescription medications can be effective. Prescribed oral medications (such as isotretinoin) and topical medications (such as benzoyl peroxide) are also available to treat acne. Usually, a combination of medications is most helpful. Not all types of acne bacteria respond to antibiotics, which can cause side effects such as yeast infections in women, light sensitivity and stomach upset.

Certain light therapies (such as blue or red light therapies prescribed by a doctor—see the section on "blue" light, below) can be helpful in treating mild to severe acne that has not responded to other treatments. This can be enhanced by adding a photo-active chemical (ALA) that enhances the penetration of the light. While mild sun exposure can lessen the redness of acne, ultraviolet rays from sunlight or a sunlamp can damage a person's skin.

Acne treatment usually needs to be continued over a long period of time, often years. Though medications used to treat acne can decrease the number of pimples or cystic lesions and prevent or stop infections, they must often be used for at least six to eight weeks before a person's skin condition starts to improve. Some treatments initially may cause a person's acne to get worse before it improves. Treatment can be expensive. People concerned about the cost of acne treatment need to talk with their health professional about ways to decrease cost. Medications for acne may cause side effects and they may stop being effective over time. Sometimes, the amount of medication used to treat acne needs to be increased to make it effective again. Surgery to remove whiteheads and blackheads or to drain pimples may be necessary.

One stalwart medication has recently come under attack. That treatment is Accutane. Although it has successfully treated acne in thousands of patients, this medication has been alleged to cause depression in some. But no medication is smart enough to do one thing and one thing only, and I personally believe this side-effect to be very rare.

Left untreated, acne can lead to scarring. Cosmetic surgery is occasionally recommended for people who have disfiguring scars due to severe acne. Needless to say, all treatment for acne scars needs to be undertaken by specially trained health professionals. Deeper scars are usually harder to treat than scars that are closer to the skin surface. Lasers, surgery, chemical peels, and filling substances are useful in this regard.

## A New Treatment for Acne

Research into photo-therapy and photo-rejuvenation has led to an innovation in the treatment of acne that uses a high-intensity blue-violet light to precisely target porphyrins, substances on the skin that surface and ductal bacterium, *propionibacterium acnes* (*P. acnes*), feeds upon. These bacteria cause 90% of inflamed blemishes. The ClearLight Acne PhotoClearing System was the first non-drug treatment device approved by the FDA to treat moderate acne. The company claims that it produces results without the side effects of traditional acne treatments: I'm able to attest that, in my office, where we use a similar device—intense pulse light (IPL) with a headpiece

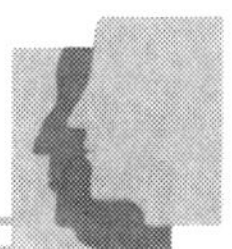

attachment and the Blu U light therapy—we attain similar results.

These devices are an exciting addition to the acne armamentarium. Patients are exposed to the light in 15-minute sessions, and the treatment regimen consists of eight sessions over a period of four weeks. A 2003 Reuters News Service report quotes Macrene Alexiades-Armenakas, MD, Ph.D., director of research at the Laser and Skin Surgery Center of New York, who is involved in clinical trials of the device. He makes the important point that this relatively passive regimen is far more likely to be followed by teenagers. His initial results in 2003 suggested that, by four weeks, there was a "significant decrease" in acne bacterial counts. He cites one published study that showed a 60% reduction in *P. acnes* counts by eight weeks and an even larger decrease of 70% after two weeks of follow-up. The results appear to be sustained and no side effects have been observed.

### *Does Diet Affect Acne?*

Recently, the American Academy of Dermatology reviewed the roll of diet in acne and concluded that two diets make acne worse in some individuals: a diet rich in refined carbohydrates (a high glycemic diet) and a diet containing lots of dairy products. Unfortunately, more research will be necessary to clarify the relationship between diet and acne.

## Eczema

Eczema is a term that describes a group of medical conditions that cause the skin to become inflamed or irritated. The most common type of eczema is known as atopic dermatitis or atopic eczema. Atopic dermatitis is the form of eczema associated with a tendency to sensitive skin. It affects about 10% to 20% of infants and about 5% to 10% of adults and children in Canada. Many infants who develop the condition outgrow it by their third birthday, while some people continue to experience symptoms on and off throughout life. But with proper treatment the disease can be controlled in the majority of sufferers.

No matter which part of the skin is affected, eczema is almost always itchy. Sometimes the itching will start before the rash appears. That's why this is known as "the itch that rashes." When the rash does appear, it most commonly occurs on the face, knees, hands, or feet, though it may also affect other areas.

Affected areas usually appear very dry, thickened, or scaly. In fair-skinned people, these areas may initially appear reddish and then turn brown. Among darker-skinned people, eczema can affect pigmentation, making the affected area lighter or darker. In infants, the itchy rash can produce an oozing, crusting condition that occurs mainly on the face and scalp, but patches may appear anywhere.

The exact cause of eczema is unknown, but it's thought to be linked to an overactive response by the body's immune system to an irritant. It is this response that causes the symptoms of the disease. In addition, eczema is commonly found in families with a history of other allergies or asthma.

Some people may suffer flare-ups of the itchy rash in response to certain substances or conditions. For some, coming into contact with rough or coarse materials may cause the skin to become itchy. For others, feeling too hot or too cold, exposure to certain household products like soap or detergent, or coming into contact with animal dander may cause an outbreak. Upper respiratory infections or colds can also be triggers, as can molds. Stress often causes the condition to worsen. Changing seasons of the year, such as spring and fall, are also problematic.

A pediatrician, dermatologist or your primary care provider can make a diagnosis of eczema. Since many people with eczema also suffer from allergies, your doctor may perform allergy tests to determine possible irritants or triggers, especially among children. Although there is no cure, most people can effectively manage their disease with medical treatment and by avoiding irritants. The condition cannot be spread from person to person.

The goal of eczema treatment is to relieve and prevent the itching

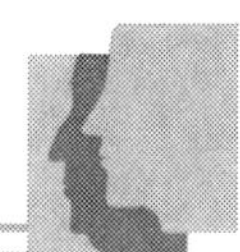

that can lead to infection. Since the disease makes skin dry and itchy, lotions and creams are recommended to keep the skin moist. These solutions are usually applied when the skin is damp—after bathing, for example—to help the skin retain moisture. Cold compresses may also be used to relieve itching.

Over-the-counter or prescription creams and ointments containing corticosteroids, such as hydrocortisone, are often prescribed to reduce inflammation. For severe cases, your doctor may prescribe oral corticosteroids. In addition, if the affected area becomes infected, your doctor may prescribe antibiotics to kill the infection-causing bacteria.

Other treatments include antihistamines to reduce severe itching, tar treatments (chemicals designed to reduce itching), phototherapy using ultraviolet light applied to the skin, and the drug cyclosporine A for people whose condition doesn't respond to other treatments.

In addition, the FDA and HPB, the drug regulatory bodies in the U.S. and Canada respectively, recently approved the first of a new class of drugs known as topical immunomodulators (TIMs) for the treatment of moderate-to-severe eczema. The drugs work by altering the immune system response to prevent flare-ups. Two of these medications are Elidel® and Protopic®. Although recently there have been questions as to their safety, dermatologists in Canada and the U.S. recognize their safety profile is excellent and most believe they should be used under certain circumstances.

Eczema outbreaks can usually be avoided or the severity lessened by following these simple tips:

- ♦ Moisturize frequently.
- ♦ Avoid sudden changes in temperature or humidity.
- ♦ Avoid sweating or overheating.
- ♦ Reduce stress.
- ♦ Avoid scratchy materials, such as wool.
- ♦ Avoid harsh soaps, detergents, and solvents.
- ♦ Avoid environmental factors that trigger allergies (for example,

pollen, mold, dust mites, and animal dander).
♦ Be aware of any foods that may cause an outbreak and avoid them.

## Melasma

Better known as "age spots" or "dark spots" related to pregnancy or hormone treatments, melasma—an area of tan or brown coloring that usually appears on the face—is a common skin condition also known as chloasma or the "mask of pregnancy." The condition occurs when the sun-exposed skin on the upper cheeks, forehead, and/or upper lip turns a tan, brownish color—the "mask"—because excess pigment is deposited in the skin's upper layers. These patches do not itch and are not red or swollen. It commonly occurs when women with skin that pigments easily, especially olive-colored skin, take oral contraceptives and very often goes away after pregnancy. In some cases, it persists and we have to try different treatments including bleaching creams or chemical peels. It's a good idea to use sunscreen during pregnancy to prevent melasma from occurring or to prevent existing patches from getting darker.

In order to lower the risk of melasma, a woman can avoid oral contraceptives and stay out of the sun and use a sunscreen with at least a 30 SPF daily. I particularly like a sunscreen known as Ti-Silc because it blocks extremely well. A healthcare provider can diagnose melasma based on its physical appearance. There are no long-term effects from melasma and treatments include:

♦ Bleaching creams
♦ Skin care products and peels that contain glycolic acid skin peels
♦ Sunscreens that extend into the UVA blocking range
♦ Fractional lasers, which help the healing process.

Side effects depend on the specific products used to treat the melasma. Some people may have a mild allergic reaction to the cream or bleach. Since the darkened skin of melasma usually fades somewhat after a woman gives birth or stops using oral contraceptives, any new

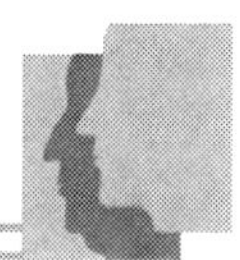

or worsening symptoms should be reported to a doctor.

Not long ago I found a few particularly effective treatment regimens known as the Obagi® and the newer Vivier Tx treatment systems. Sold only through qualified physicians, these formulations actively treat and control melasma in 90% to 95% of patients who use it. Also effective for this problem is the Cosmelan treatment.

Another treatment option is microdermabrasion and Beta-lift peels. Still another is the AFA/clay mask from Excel Cosmeceuticals, by which a clay mask is first put on, then amino acid filaggrin-based antioxidants (AFA) are applied. This patented process speeds up the removal of pigment and sun damage. It is also useful for acne.

Yet another treatment for melasma is fractional resurfacing. The equipment produces a distinctive thermal damage pattern by creating discrete columns of thermal damage referred to as microthermal treatment zones. It characteristically spares the tissue surrounding each microthermal treatment zone, and seems to lead to faster epidermal repair. Fractional resurfacing has been successfully used in treating not just melasma, but dyschromia, lentigenes, wrinkles, and acne scars. It offers minimal downtime but is safer to use off the face and on darker skin types.

## Rosacea

Sometimes known as the red mask, this is a condition gaining more notoriety lately. Some people may notice that their skin has become very sensitive before they begin to notice symptoms of rosacea. For example, they may notice that facial products burn their skin.

Rosacea is usually first noticed when redness on the cheeks lingers, similar to a slight sunburn. This redness and other symptoms of rosacea come and go. However, with time, the symptoms become persistent.

The main symptoms include:

- Redness on the face. The redness is caused by flushing when a sudden increase of blood flows through the blood vessels, and the blood vessels expand. Redness usually appears in women on the cheeks, nose, chin, and forehead. The redness may appear in a "butterfly" distribution across the cheeks and nose. Facial redness in men typically appears on the nose, although symptoms can appear in other areas of the face. In some cases, redness may also occur on the neck and upper chest.

♦ Pimples on the face. Small pimples may occur on the red areas of skin or on the edges. These pimples—red, round bumps in the skin—are different from acne pimples, which have blackheads or whiteheads.

♦ Red lines on the face. Small, thin red lines, which are tiny blood vessels with a spider-like appearance, may be noticed on the face, usually on the cheeks. This condition is called telangiectasia.

♦ Swollen red bumps on the nose. These are underground pimples that don't come to a head. In severe cases, mostly in men, the nose appears enlarged, bulbous, and red, a condition called rhinophyma.

♦ Irritation in the eye. Symptoms in the eye include redness, dryness, burning, presence of crusted mucus, tearing, a gritty sensation (like that of sand in the eye), pinkeye (conjunctivitis), and swelling in the eyelid. There may be intolerance for contact lenses, and styes may develop.

About half of the people who have rosacea may have some eye irritation or symptoms. In some severe cases, vision may become blurry.

People who have rosacea may get migraine headaches more often than people who do not have this condition. Rosacea is a chronic condition, with symptoms that come and go with frequent flare-ups. The goal of treatment for rosacea is to reduce or eliminate symptoms and stop the condition from getting worse. Presently, there is no cure for rosacea. Treatment is usually successful in minimizing symptoms, and preventing disease progression and severe complications, especially if started when symptoms are first noticed. If untreated, rosacea symptoms—redness, small red lines, and pimples—can get worse, recur

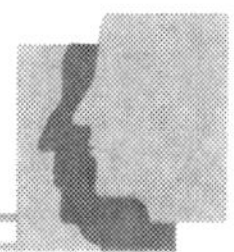

more often, and eventually become permanent.

Symptoms of the three main forms of rosacea vary and may require different treatment.

♦ Papulopustular form. Small pimples, or papules, develop on the face. These red, round bumps in the skin are different from acne pimples. Topical and oral antibiotics are generally prescribed for the early stages of rosacea, including general redness of the face. In severe cases, dermabrasion surgery may be performed.

♦ Telangiectatis form. Small, thin red lines, which are tiny blood vessels with a spider-like appearance, develop on the face, usually on the cheeks. If antibiotics are not effective in treating this form of rosacea, your doctor may suggest laser surgery using a pulsed-dye laser (also called "intense pulse light" or "IPL treatment").

♦ Granulomatous form. Swollen bumps occur on the nose and cheeks. If the condition becomes severe, chronic inflammation may cause the nose to look enlarged, bulbous, and red. This condition is called rhinophyma. This type of rosacea usually does not respond to antibiotic treatment. Various surgical procedures, such as dermabrasion, laser resurfacing , and cosmetic surgery, may improve the effects of granulmatous rosacea and enlargement of the nose.

With antibiotic treatment, rosacea symptoms usually improve in three to four months, with greater improvement occurring in six months to a year. In addition to antibiotics, identifying and avoiding triggers that cause flare-ups is important to the success of treatment. By keeping a list or diary to identify triggers, people can avoid those foods, products, or activities that might cause flare-ups. Even people who are using medication to control rosacea benefit from avoiding triggers.

The success of surgery depends on your skin type and condition, your doctor's level of experience, the type of surgery used, your lifestyle, and amount of sun exposure following the procedure. Some types of skin problems respond better to surgery than others. Surgery may also be used to reduce general redness of the face.

Three very important treatments are often overlooked. The first is to use creams containing vitamin C, which stabilize blood vessels. A second is to use creams and peels that contain amino fruit acids (AFA). A third is the use of IPLs and vascular lasers, with or without ALA. Finally, cover-ups, especially mineral-based makeup such as Glominerals, help to hide problems while they heal and sunscreens help to prevent flare-ups.

### Milia

Unlike many of the conditions described here, milia can occur in babies as well as adults. The condition produces tiny white spots appearing on the face of a newborn as a result of unopened oil (sebaceous) glands. In adults, it is due to glands being plugged. Milia usually disappear spontaneously within a few weeks, but more serious cases can be treated with topical creams such as vitamin A, the AFA/clay mask or, in extreme cases, microdermabrasion.

### Seborrheic Keratoses

A form of "age spots," which I prefer to call "maturing spots" or "wisdom spots," this condition produces rough, waxy brown or black spots. They may start appearing on your skin just before midlife and become increasingly prevalent with age. Flat, brown spots that form after years of sun exposure—age spots, also called "solar lentigines"—are common in adults who have tanned or spent a lot of time outdoors. The best treatment for this condition is prevention—wearing the appropriate sun block throughout your youth and adulthood. The second best is good skin care with the Obagi® or Vivier Tx products accompanied by regular microdermabrasion or AFA/clay peels. The third best is liquid nitrogen and/or lasers to treat these unsightly lesions.

### Age Spots vs. Cancer

How do you know the difference between simple age spots and possible skin cancer? As an MD, I recommend that you visit your health

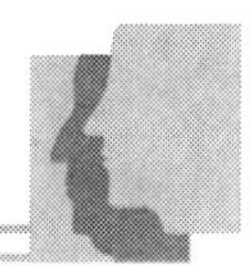

care professional for an accurate diagnosis. Mole-like spots can appear on your skin at any age, and while many of these spots may be harmless, you should keep an eye out for signs of cancer.

How do you separate harmless moles from potentially cancerous ones? Check for the ABCDEs:

◆ A is for asymmetry. This means that if you divide the mole in half, the two parts do not match. Asymmetry may be a sign of cancer.

◆ B is for border. Irregular edges that are ragged or notched may be a suspicious sign.

◆ C is for color. Uneven or multiple colors that may vary from brown, black, and pink to red, white, and blue can signal melanoma, a type of skin cancer that can be deadly.

◆ D is for diameter. A mole may be abnormal if it is bigger than a pencil eraser.

◆ E is for elevation. A raised or uneven mole can be a sign of skin cancer.

If a skin marking has any of the characteristics listed above, your doctor should evaluate it as soon as possible.

Also look for other warning signs of skin cancer, including a mole that appears to be new or growing; changes in appearance or texture, itches, hurts, or feels different than usual; or is crusted, swollen, red, or irritated.

No matter what has caused your spots, the best way to detect any changes in your skin is to give yourself a monthly full-body skin self-exam and to see your health care professional regularly for a thorough skin exam. According to the American Cancer Society, these exams should be done every three years between the ages of 20 and 39 and yearly starting at age 40. You may need more frequent exams if you've had skin cancer in the past. And, of course, promptly contact your doctor's office anytime you detect a growth that looks suspicious or worries you.

## Keratosis Pilaris

This ailment has a silly nickname, but it can be an embarrassing matter to those who suffer from it. Also known as "chicken skin," keratosis pilaris is a common, harmless skin condition. These rough, goose-bumpy, sandpaper-like patches are usually seen on the backs of the arms and outer thighs but can show up anywhere hair grows.

Sometimes keratosis pilaris is confused with pimples or ingrown hairs. But whereas the bumps in such conditions vary in size, shape, and arrangement, keratosis pilaris is uniform. The lesions are generally the same in appearance and form a regular pattern.

This condition is caused by rough follicular papules—in other words, the top layer of skin where the hair emerges is jagged and upraised. It is often associated with atopic dermatitis (also called eczema), which is characterized by red, itchy skin patches, but it can also be seen alone. Keratosis pilaris tends to run in families and most frequently occurs in children and teens. Most people simply grow out of it in their late 20s or early 30s.

You're on the right track with the lotion and loofah sponge, but those won't get rid of the problem. What's more, vigorous scrubbing may make the area more inflamed. Follow these steps to minimize the appearance of the bumps:

♦ Ask your doctor for a urea cream (like Uremol®20) and ask your doctor to get the pharmacist to mix it with 2% to 3% salicylic acid. Uremol 20 is available by prescription from your pharmacy.

♦ After showering, gently pat the skin dry, leaving the affected areas slightly moist.

♦ Rub the cream on the affected areas and gently buff with a loofah for five seconds.

♦ If your skin shows no sign of irritation after a week, increase the buffing time by five seconds a week until you reach 20 seconds per area. Don't exceed the recommended buffing time, as it won't make the condition go away faster and could cause further irritation.

♦ Once the bumps are under control, you can reduce the buffing to

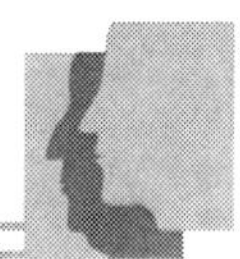

once or twice a week and use plain urea cream, *without* the added salicylic acid.

If the condition doesn't diminish or gets worse after following these instructions for a few weeks, see a dermatologist.

## Scars & Scar Treatments

### Scars

Whether caused by teenage acne, surgery, accidents, burns or sports injuries, scars are now a correctable condition. But, which of the techniques we've already discussed is best to reduce their appearance? Chemical peels? Dermabrasion? Laser resurfacing? You've begun looking for ways to improve the acne scars on your face or the surgical scar on your leg, what's the best option for you?

Laser resurfacing may hold promise as a new treatment for scars, but according to a recent report in the *British Journal of Dermatology* (BJD), patients need more information before making a choice.

### Acne Scars

Dermatologists have been using lasers to treat scarring for a number of years. One is the Ultrapulse $C0_2$ laser, which produces excellent results even though it takes a little while to heal. After surgery, patients apply a special dressing and see the doctor regularly. The treated skin is swollen and irritated at first, as though it were a bad sunburn, but it recovers within two weeks. With this rapid healing, new skin is laid down and scars generally improve.

The BJD reviewed 16 research studies on laser resurfacing for facial acne scars. There were no standard measures for scar improvement or patient satisfaction, but the findings suggest that the procedure is up to 90% effective and is more precise than dermabrasion (in which a rough, abrasive diamond fraise is used to remove scars), and chemical peels (in which chemicals remove layers of skin).

Lasers are named according to the source that creates the energy beam. For example, erbium lasers use erbium gases to produce energy. Certain lasers are more useful for certain procedures and certain skin types. For example, the erbium YAG laser is better for improving darker skin because it penetrates less deeply. Most of the studies the BJD looked at tested the effectiveness of the carbon dioxide laser, although results were similar with the YAG laser. In all cases, a new skin surface formed within 10 days, and redness lasted for about two months. Up to 45% of the patients had temporary changes in skin color, but infections were rare.

Dermatologists say outcomes are determined by scar depth and patient expectations. Laser resurfacing is most effective for shallow scars that can be stretched with the fingers. Patients can usually expect a 50% to 80% improvement but should allow 18 months for complete remodeling after a procedure. Deep or "ice pick" acne scars can be treated in several ways before or during laser resurfacing.

Recently, a new type of laser has come to the forefront for treating scars. It is known as fractional resurfacing and it uses a laser to treat damaged and aging skin by harmlessly penetrating the outer layer of skin, but only resurfacing 15 to 20% of the skin during each session. This method protects the skin from sustaining too much damage at once and eliminates much of the downtime associated with $CO_2$ or erbium laser resurfacing treatment. Several companies make lasers of this type. Their main drawback is that treatment must be repeated several times for optimal results.

Full-face laser resurfacing presently ranges between $6,000 and $10,000, with fractional resurfacing costing $500 to $2,000 a treatment But even with the out-of-pocket cost, these are still good options. Downtime and inconvenience are nothing compared to the benefits of scar reduction, because having more confidence improves just about everything.

## Surgical Scarring

Meanwhile, surgical scars are becoming less of an issue. Operations that once meant a lengthy hospital stay, a long and painful recovery period and permanent scarring may now be less painful, virtually scar-free, and require much less time in a hospital bed—all thanks to a new technique called "needlescopic" (or "endoscopic") surgery. This is the technique by which a camera is inserted through a small tube and used to scope the digestive organs. It has also found application in other surgeries, although of course intestinal surgery and face surgery require different types of tubes.

The point of these less invasive types of surgery such as needlescopic (and the older, more familiar laparascopic, which use small incisions, small surgical tools, and a telescope-like instrument, is to diminish the trauma to the abdominal wall so patients have less pain, smaller scars, and recover more quickly.

In needlescopic surgery, the size of the instruments is reduced from the 5 to 12 mm diameter of standard laparoscopic surgery to less than 3 mm. Because needlescopic instruments are so fine and sharp, there was some concern that they might increase the threat of organ perforations. In fact doctors see no difference in complication rates between needlescopic and laparoscopic surgery, and needlescopic surgery means shorter hospital stays.

Most surgeons know intuitively who is and isn't a good candidate for needlescopic surgery. Nonetheless, the technology does have limitations, and there are some basic caveats. At the present time, big people, big organs, and major gastrointestinal surgeries are difficult to deal with by needlescopic surgery. The development of sturdier instruments may change things, but for now the bottom line is that obese patients are not good candidates, and this does not work for removing heavy, enlarged organs, because the instruments may break. In the right patient, however, needlescopic surgery is an attractive option. Doctors can offer needlescopic surgery to some patients with the understanding that they might have to switch to standard instruments during the operation. In the middle of the procedure, if there is difficulty, the surgeon can change to larger instruments or even to traditional open surgery.

# Chapter 3

# Your Face

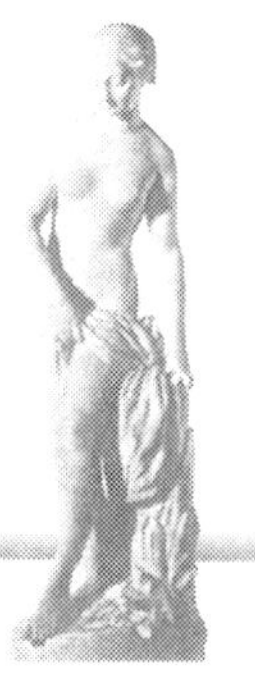

Only a small portion of our skin covers our face, but for us humans, it is a most important part. The face—the front of our head—holds most of our sensory organs and is normally exposed at all times. We have evolved an acute ability to differentiate these highly visible faces from one another and so identify other individuals instantly. Perhaps it is this refined sensitivity to facial differences that has led us to endow our perceptions of the face with intense characteristics of beauty and ugliness: we judge the face more sharply than any other part of the body. On the other hand, just because the face *must* be exposed to the world, it is most vulnerable to the destructive forces in our environment.

## *Wrinkles*

While many people believe wrinkles are somehow a sign of authority or wisdom, there can be no doubt they're also a sign of aging. The good news is that you don't have to put up with them, and the first step is to understand them and know from where they come.

Wrinkles are a by-product of the aging process. With age, skin cells divide more slowly, and the inner layer, the dermis, begins to thin. The networks of elastin (the protein that causes skin to stretch) and collagen fibers (the major structural proteins in the skin) that support the outer layer, loosen and unravel, eventually causing depressions on the surface. As the skin loses its elasticity it's less able to retain moisture. Oil-secreting glands are less efficient and the skin is slower to heal. The skin's hyaluronic acid also slowly decreases. All of these contribute to the development of wrinkles.

Lines between the eyebrows (frown lines) and lines jutting from the corner of the eyes (crow's feet) are believed to develop because of loosening and drooping of the skin and small muscle contractions. Smiling, frowning, squinting and other habitual facial expressions cause these wrinkles to become more prominent. Over time, these expressions, coupled with gravity, contribute to the formation of jowls , drooping eyelids and smile lines.

Again, exposure to the sun's ultraviolet radiation can result in the premature aging of skin called "photo-aging." The sun's ultraviolet rays damage collagen fibers and cause the excessive production of abnormal elastin. When ultraviolet light damages skin tissue, an enzyme called metalloproteinase is produced. This enzyme creates and reforms collagen. During the process, however, some healthy collagen fibers are damaged, resulting in a disorganized formation of fibers called solar comedones. Wrinkles develop when the rebuilding process occurs repeatedly.

The sun's rays make us feel good and in the short term produces vitamin D and give us a sense of vitality. But our love of the sun isn't reciprocated: exposure to the sun causes most of the wrinkles that haunt our faces.

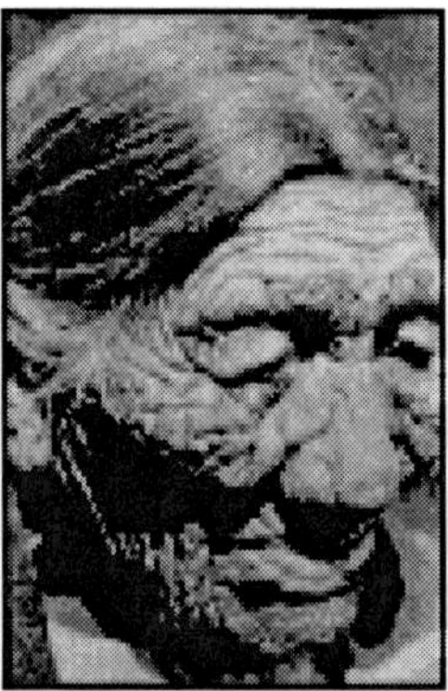

A Pueblo Indian woman with a lifetime of exposure to the sun.

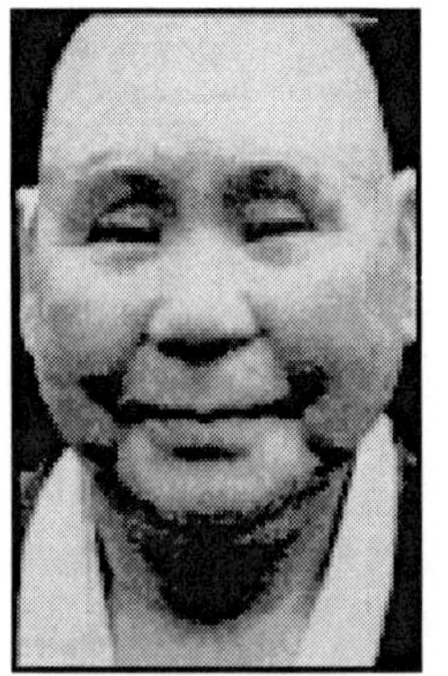

A Buddhist monk with little exposure to the sun.

Photos courtesy of Al Kligman

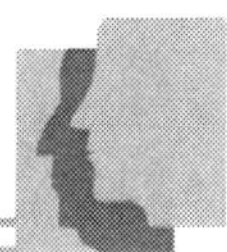

These two pictures are my favorite illustrations of the power of the sun.

The picture on the right is a Buddhist monk, age 80. He has stayed in a monastery since he was a boy and has seen little sunlight. His skin looks like a baby's, without a single wrinkle or blemish.

The picture on the left is of a 53-year-old Pueblo Indian from the desert of New Mexico. Having lived in the sun all her life, her skin is severely wrinkled: a roadmap of experience—and the record of decades of sunshine.

If you doubt this, you can see the effects of the sun on your own skin. Look at your arms. Then, in a mirror, look at the skin of your buttocks. The protected skin is smoother and softer.

Healthy skin perpetually regenerates but smoking can interfere in this process. While old collagen is broken down and removed, new collagen is produced. Researchers have found that smoke causes a marked reduction in the production of new collagen. A lack of new collagen results in the development of wrinkles.

But apart from avoiding over-exposure to the sun and cigarette smoke, what can you do to treat wrinkles as they arise?

Removing skin layers to reduce wrinkles or irregular depressions is an effective way to regain smoother, more youthful looking skin. Microdermabrasion (scraping layers away) and chemical peels (dissolving skin away) are two of the well-established methods used in skin resurfacing. Aside from these procedures, several newer techniques have been developed:

♦ Laser skin-resurfacing. The laser can do the same job as that done by microdermabrasion and chemical peels, and sometimes do it better. An erbium or carbon dioxide laser can help limit the downtime after a laser procedure and the results can last for years. A new variant, the Arctic® peel, uses an erbium laser to precisely remove the epidermis and results in further reduction of downtime.

♦ Botox procedures are injections that remove wrinkles by affecting the muscles acting on loose skin.

♦ Photorejuvenation with intense pulse light (IPL) attacks pigmented changes associated with aging. Recently, an adaptation known as aminolevulinic acid/photodynamic therapy (ALA/PDT), which uses the ALA as a photo-enhancer, increases the efficacy of the light and decreases the number of treatments necessary.

If you are considering treatment for your wrinkles, ask your dermatologist which procedure is right for you. There is no replacement for your dermatologist's professional advice because a dermatologist is a trained and experienced skin expert. Your dermatologist can recommend a therapy tailored individually to your skin's requirements

## Preventing Wrinkles

You may have been noticing the signs of aging for a while: increased roughness, wrinkling, irregular pigmentation (coloration) or inelasticity. These are all normal changes in our skin as we age.

You may have enlarged sebaceous (oil) glands. These are often shown as little yellow bumps on your skin and have a characteristic central depression.

Sometimes, pre-cancerous and cancerous lesions can occur with aged and photo-aged skin. Knowing how to differentiate between these and benign conditions can save your life.

Our skin doesn't produce new cells at the same pace as we age and requires more care than younger skin. Environmental and biological factors take their toll. Often we develop enlarged pores, and the effects of the sun become evident in sunspots, freckles and wrinkles.

Here are three tips to enhance natural skin care as you grow older: Seek out skin-care products such as creams that help you manage your skin cells. Look for products that contain ingredients such as vitamin B complex, copper, flax oil, hydroquinone, vitamin C and glycolic acid. More recently, biological growth factors have been added to the list to optimize results.

♦ If you smoke, stop. Smoking has been shown to accelerate aging of skin, so quitting now is important for good skin health. Ask your

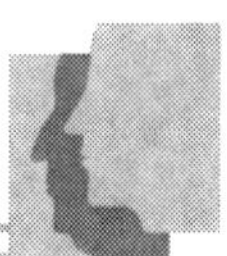

family doctor for techniques to help break this habit.

♦ A well-balanced diet—with or without a multivitamin—helps the skin get the nutrition it needs to help repair ongoing damage from the sun and other environmental elements. Drink a lot of water to hydrate your skin from the inside out.

Many topical non-prescription and prescription products that help maintain and protect your skin's health are currently available. Ask your doctor or skin-care specialist which medications are best for you.

## Antioxidants

Antioxidant supplements and specialized skin-care products are now popular treatments for the slowing of aging and prevention of wrinkles and other unpleasant side-effects of aging such as spots, stiff joints and fatigue. But as more people join the ranks of older population, they're finding that staying young isn't always as simple as taking a few pills and smearing on special lotions. Geneticists tell us that this is because the cause of aging goes much deeper, all the way into the core of the body's cells—the genes—the blueprints of human life that dictate how people grow, develop and age.

There are many genes that may play a role in how we age and how long we live, as demonstrated in extreme cases like Werner's Syndrome, a disease that causes people to develop symptoms of aging as early as age twenty. Persons with the syndrome develop gray hair, osteoporosis, heart disease and diabetes—symptoms that often mar the health of an aging person. In 1996, doctors isolated the cause: a gene they call recQ, mutated so that it no longer works to support the cell's gene-maintenance machinery. When the machine slows down, the person affected begins to display the signs of premature aging. Because an alteration in a single gene causes symptoms of aging, physicians might someday be able to target certain normal genes to slow the aging process.

More clues have emerged from the study of animals whose genes are similar to human genes. Scientists have found several genes in roundworms, for example, that when mutated allow the worms to live twice as long. One of these genes controls how much antioxidant the body produces. When the gene is mutated, more antioxidant is produced to fight free radicals, by-products of the body's energy-making process that cause aging by damaging tissues and cells. Roundworms that have more of the antioxidant live twice as long as worms that have the normal amount of antioxidant.

One of the most potent of these antioxidants is vitamin C (L-ascorbic acid). Humans do not produce vitamin C internally and therefore require dietary or supplemental sources of this vitamin. High concentrations of vitamin C in formulations for skin-care (5% and 10% creams and solutions) have been difficult and challenging to manufacture and once manufactured, difficult to keep stable. Vitamin C has tended to oxidize and turn a yellowish-brown color and for this reason, some manufacturers have avoided stating the vitamin C concentration values on their labels and packaging. Others have manufactured vitamin C products at significantly lower concentrations. But to be effective in skin-care products, vitamin C concentrations must be in the range of 5% to 10%. Two advances have now made vitamin C a viable cosmetic product. First, the vitamin has been stabilized. This is important because older formulations used to break down before they could positively affect the skin. The second development is delivery systems that carry vitamin into the skin. According to the promotional material for one of these products—the IntraDermal System™ from Vivier Pharma Inc.—IDS™ controls penetration for a longer lasting effect, has a reduced systemic effect with a broad and flexible applicability, is a simple cost-effect formulation with good stability, sustained action and increased therapeutic effect. They claim that the compound has ability to "increase drug flux across the stratum corneum (the true skin) by diffusion and thereby changing the ability of the drug to penetrate the intercellular space…in the layers of the skin (stratum corneum, epidermis and dermis)."

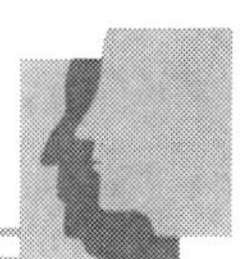

## CARING FOR YOUR FACE: PRODUCTS

### KNOWING YOUR SKIN

When you're researching over-the-counter skin-care products, the most important thing to remember is to trust yourself. No one knows your skin better than you do. There are many skin-care products on the market and it's easy to waste a lot of time and money trying to find the best solution by trial and error. Take a minute to educate yourself before making your purchases. And remember, this information I'm going to give you in this section is only a guide. Check with your dermatologist or physician if you have specific problems with your skin.

There are a few basic questions about your skin that you should ask.

- Your skin type. It is oily, dry, normal, sensitive, or a combination?
- Your skin complexion. Do you have fair skin that sunburns easily or
- Light to medium skin that may also sunburn?
- A medium tone that usually tans?
- A darker complexion that only rarely burns?
- Is your complexion so dark that you never burn?

Here is a little table that shows the skin types.

This important table tells you how your skin will react to the sun. For example, if you are type one and always burn, you must consciously take steps to avoid the sun. You must use a high-powered sunscreen and avoid the sun, especially at midday when it is most intense.

### Your Skin Concerns

Are you looking for a program of preventative maintenance to avoid premature aging? Do you have a skin problem, such as persistent acne, age spots, melasma or rosacea? Do you have large pores, sun damage, facial wrinkles or fine lines that require special attention? Do you have eye puffiness or under-eye bags that will require special

| Fitzpatrick Classification of Sun Reactive Skin Types | | |
|---|---|---|
| Skin Type | Color | Reaction to the Sun |
| I | White | Always burns, never tans |
| II | White | Sometimes burns but tans with difficulty |
| III | White | Sometimes burns but tans easily |
| IV | Moderate brown | Rarely burns, tans very easily |
| V | Dark brown | Very rarely burns, most often tans |
| VI | Black | Never burns, always tans |

care? Are you a smoker? Do you spend a lot of time in the sun? Do you take a daily vitamin? Do you consume a well-balanced diet?

When you've answered those questions, you'll be better equipped to wisely sort through skin-care products to find the ones suited to your specific skin type. If you need further help, ask your cosmetic doctor or a specially trained esthetician at a medical spa for his or her recommendations.

To assist you during that process, here is some information about skin-care chemistry and the latest ingredients in products that may benefit your skin. Use it to sort through the various skin-care products on the market.

## Alpha-Hydroxy Acids (AHAs)

Over-the-counter skin-care products containing alpha-hydroxy acids (glycolic, lactic, tartaric and citric acids) have become increasingly popular over the last five years. In the U.S. alone, there are over 200 manufacturers of skin-care products containing these acids. Creams

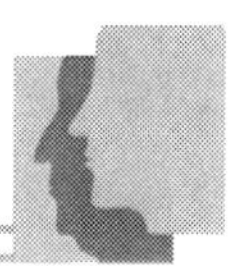

and lotions with alpha-hydroxy acids may help with fine lines, irregular pigmentation and age spots, and may help decrease enlarged pores. Side effects of alpha-hydroxy acids include mild irritation and sun sensitivity. For that reason, sunscreen also should be used with AHA every morning. To help avoid skin irritation with alpha-hydroxy acids, I suggest you start with a product with mild concentrations of AHA (10 to15%) Also, make sure you ease into it. You want to get your skin used to alpha-hydroxy acids, so you should only initially apply these products every other day, then gradually work up to daily application.

## Beta-hydroxy Acid (Salicylic Acid)

Salicylic acid also has been studied for its effect on skin that has aged prematurely due to exposure to ultraviolet rays from the sun. This acid exfoliates skin, that is, it removes the top layer of skin cells and can improve the texture and color of the skin. It penetrates and opens oil-laden hair follicle openings and, as a result, also helps with acne.

In higher concentrations (20% to 30%) salicylic acid works well as a peel to treat acne and hyperpigmentation. A peel is a very strong exfoliant process that affects the top layer(s) of the skin. I find the product called "Beta-lift" peel particularly useful.

Some skin-care products that contain salicylic acid are available over the counter and others require a doctor's prescription. Studies have shown that salicylic acid is less irritating than skin-care products containing alpha-hydroxy acids, while providing similar improvement in skin texture and color.

## Hydroquinone

Products containing hydroquinone are popularly referred to as "bleaching creams" or "lightening agents." These skin care products are used to lighten hyperpigmentation, such as age spots and dark spots related to pregnancy or hormone therapy (melasma or chloasma). Some over-the-counter skin care products contain hydroquinone, but your doctor can also prescribe a solution with a higher concentration of hydroquinone if your skin doesn't respond to over-the-counter treatments. I've found 95% of my patients with increased pigment (melasma) will respond to hydroquinone used in the Obagi® skin protocols or Vivier Tx program. If you are allergic to hydroquinones, you can use products containing kojic acid instead.

## Kojic Acid

Kojic acid is a more recent remedy for the treatment of pigment problems and age spots. Discovered in 1989, kojic acid has an effect similar to hydroquinone, but it is less potent. Kojic acid is derived from a fungus, and studies have shown that it is effective as a lightening agent, inhibiting production of melanin (brown pigment).

## Retinol

You'll notice that many skin-care products contain retinol, a derivative of vitamin A. Retinol's stronger counterpart is tretinoin, a prescription agent that is the active ingredient in Retin-A®, and Renova®. And most recently I've found two other agents that work well: tazarotene (Tazorac®) and adapalene (Differin®). If your skin is too sensitive to use Retin-A, retinol is a good alternative. Skin responds to products that contain retinol because vitamin A has a molecular structure that's tiny enough to get into the lower layers of skin, where it stimulates the formation of collage and elastin. It also helps normalize the epidermis, allowing the skin to return to an appearance it had before sun exposure. Retinol is proven to improve mottled pigmentation, fine lines and wrinkles, skin texture, skin tone and color, and dry skin's low hydration levels.

You may also hear about retinyl palmitate. This falls into the same family as retinol, but, to get the same effect, you'll need to use more of a product that contains retinyl palmitate than one that contains retinol.

### L-Ascorbic Acid

We discussed vitamin C earlier in the section on sun damage. L-ascorbic acid is the only form of vitamin C that you should consider for your skin. There are many products on the market today that boast vitamin C derivatives (magnesium ascorbyl phosphate or ascorbyl palmitate, for example) as ingredients, but L-ascorbic acid appears to be the only form of vitamin C useful for skin-care. Vitamin C is also the only antioxidant that is proven to stimulate the synthesis of collagen. This is essential since your body's natural collagen production decreases as you age. Sun exposure will also accelerate the decrease in collagen. Studies have shown that vitamin C helps to minimize fine lines, scars, and wrinkles.

### Hyaluronic Acid

Skin-care products containing this substance are often used in conjunction with vitamin C products to assist in effective penetration. Hyaluronic acid (also known as a glycosaminoglycan) is often touted for its ability to "reverse" or "stop" aging. You might have heard hyaluronic acid referred to in the media as a "key factor in youth." This is because the substance occurs naturally (and quite abundantly) in humans and animals, where it is a component of the body's connective tissues, and is known to cushion and lubricate. It is found in young skin, and in other tissues such as the eye and joint fluid. As you age, however, various natural factors destroy hyaluronic acid. Diet and smoking can also affect your body's level of hyaluronic acid over time. Skin-care products with hyaluronic acid are most frequently used to treat wrinkled skin.

### Copper Peptide

Copper peptide is often referred to as the most effective skin regeneration product, even though it's only been on the market since 1997. Studies have shown that copper peptide promotes collagen and elastin production, acts as an antioxidant and promotes production of glycosaminoglycans such as hyaluronic acid. It appears that copper-dependent enzymes increase the benefits of the body's natural tissue-building processes. The substance helps to firm, smooth, and soften skin, doing it in less time than most other anti-aging products. Clinical studies have found that copper peptides also remove damaged collagen and elastin from the skin and scar tissue because they activate the skin's system responsible for those functions.

### Alpha-Lipoic Acid

You may have heard of alpha-lipoic acid as "the miracle in a jar" for its anti-aging effects. It's a newer, ultra-potent antioxidant that helps fight future skin damage and helps repair past damage. Alpha-lipoic acid has been referred to as a "universal antioxidant" because it's soluble in both water and oil, which allows it access to all parts of the skin cell. For this reason, many researchers believe that alpha-lipoic acid can provide the greatest protection against damaging free radicals when compared with other antioxidants. Alpha-lipoic acid diminishes fine lines, gives skin a healthy glow and boosts levels of other antioxidants such as vitamin C.

### DMAE (Dimethylaminoethanol)

Fish is often referred to as brain food, and for this we can thank DMAE. This substance—naturally produced in the brain but also present in anchovies, salmon and sardines—stimulates the production of acetylcholine, which is important for proper mental functions. DMAE in skin-care products can show remarkable effects when applied topically to skin, resulting in a reduction of fine lines and wrinkles.

### Biological Growth Factors

If you could apply a safe, natural nutrient solution to your skin in 30 seconds, twice a day and look younger in 90 days, would you do it?

Skin Medica Inc. promotes its SkinMedica TNS Recovery

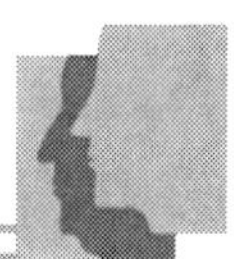

Complex with NouriCel-MD, a bioengineered product using sophisticated biological growth factors, as able to achieve these results, visible in as little as one week. Scientific studies have shown measurably younger-looking skin with improved elasticity and a decrease in age spots and pigmentation within 90 days. Oprah Winfrey featured the product.

NouriCel-MD is a new product that provides an alternative to current skin care regimens. It contains topical human-growth factors that are derived through a patented process. Its proteins appear to improve the appearance of aging and sun-damaged skin. In addition to topical human growth factors, it contains antioxidants, soluble collagens and proteins—compounds produced by healthy new skin.

## Summary

Researchers continue to develop innovations in skin rejuvenation that range from topically applied "cosmeceuticals" to the new surgical techniques we'll come to shortly. A thorough understanding of how your skin changes as you age and how the sun affects your skin can help you and your doctor decide what treatment is suited for you.

But remember, the best way to keep skin healthy is to avoid sun exposure beginning early in life. Here are some other tips:

- Do not sunbathe or visit tanning parlors and try to stay out of the sun between 10 A.M. and 3 P.M.
- If you are in the sun between 10 A.M. and 3 P.M., always wear protective clothing such as a hat, long-sleeved shirt, and sunglasses.
- Put on sunscreen lotion before going out in the sun to help protect your skin from UV light. Remember to reapply the lotion as needed. Always use products that are SPF (sun protection factor) 15 or higher. I personally prefer 30 or higher.
- Check your skin often for signs of skin cancer. If there are changes that worry you, call the doctor right away. The American Academy of Dermatology suggests that older, fair-skinned people have a

yearly skin check by a doctor as part of a regular physical check-up.
♦ Relieve dry-skin problems by using a humidifier at home, bathing with soap less often (use a moisturizing body wash instead), and using a moisturizing lotion. If this doesn't work, see your doctor.

## Caring for Your Face: Special Procedures

For most of us, whether we like it or not, the size, shape, and look of our bodies influences how we see ourselves, how others see us and, in some cases, how we function. There is nothing wrong with wanting to change the way you look. Just as some people choose to do this through diet, exercise, and other lifestyle changes, others may choose to have cosmetic surgery, especially if they are unhappy with a specific aspect of their body or appearance that surgery could alter.

However, the decision to have cosmetic surgery should not be taken lightly. Surgery always involves some level of risk. Complications can occur. There is no guarantee that you will get the results you want. If you are considering the surgical option, make sure that you measure the possible benefits of cosmetic surgery against the possible problems or dangers that could result from surgery.

For people who are unhappy with their overall appearance rather than just a specific aspect of their appearance, cosmetic surgery is probably not the answer. They are unlikely to be satisfied with the results of a single cosmetic surgery procedure and may fall into a pattern of having one procedure after another. This can be risky, damaging to the body, and quite costly. It is very important to have realistic expectations about how cosmetic surgery may or may not affect your life. Appearance is only a small part of who a person is.

There is no clear line to be drawn between cosmetic "treatments," cosmetic "procedures" and cosmetic "surgery." Everything we have said above can apply to any of them. However, for the purposes of our discussion of the face, we will look first at the less invasive "procedures" and then at the more "aggressive" surgical techniques. Then

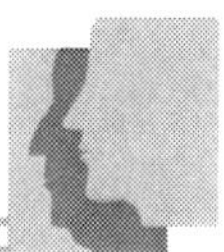

we'll cover some of these in more details in *The Body* chapter.

## Chemical Peels

Chemical peeling is a skin resurfacing process that uses a chemical solution to remove the top layers of skin, allowing new skin to grow. It is most often used to remove wrinkles, superficial skin growths, shallow scars, pigment changes in the skin, and other skin problems.

A chemical peel is applied to the skin and allowed to penetrate it. The skin then peels off over a period of one to fourteen days, depending on how deeply the chemical penetrated the skin. This procedure destroys parts of the skin in a controlled way so that new skin can grow in its place. The chemicals used are sometimes called exfoliating or wounding agents.

Chemical peels are classified according to how deeply the chemical penetrates and what type of chemical solution is used. Factors that may affect the depth of a peel include the acid concentration of the peeling agent, the number of coats that are applied, and the amount of time allowed before the acid is neutralized. Deeper peels result in more dramatic effects as well as higher risks, increased pain, and longer healing time. Before the peel, your doctor can help you decide what depth of peel and what type of chemical solution is most appropriate, based on your skin type, which areas you want peeled, what kind of results you want, how much risk you are willing to take, and other issues. A small "test spot" may be peeled to get a better idea of the results, especially for people with darker skin.

### *Types of Peel*

There are three basic types of peels.

- Superficial peels are used to improve the appearance of pigment changes in the skin, acne scars, mild sun damage, or fine wrinkles in all skin types. They can be done on the face and on other parts of the body. A superficial peel may also be used to prepare the skin for a deeper peel. Superficial peels are the mildest type of chemical peel and can be used on all skin types. Superficial peels usually use liquid containing a mild (dilute) acid, most often glycolic acid. Dry ice (solid carbon dioxide) is sometimes used.

♦ Medium peels are used to treat mild to moderate wrinkles, long-term sun damage, pigment changes, and precancerous lesions of the skin (usually caused by sun exposure). Medium peels are used most often on the face. Medium peels penetrate the skin more deeply than superficial peels and cause a second-degree burn of the skin. Trichloroacetic acid (TCA) is the main peeling agent used for medium peels, though the peel may also be done in several steps using a different chemical solution followed by TCA.

♦ Deep peels are used to treat severe wrinkles, long-term sun damage, pronounced pigment changes, and lesions and growths of the skin. They are done only on the face and penetrate several layers of skin and cause a second-degree burn of the skin. A chemical called phenol is usually used for a deep peel. Deep peels may not be used on darker skin types because they tend to bleach the skin (hypopigmentation). Even in lighter-skinned people, phenol peels—or any type of deep resurfacing—may cause hypopigmentation. A deep peel can be done only once in most cases.

### *Preparation*

Two to three weeks before the peel, you will need to begin preparing your skin by cleansing it twice a day, applying a special moisturizer or cream once or twice a day, and using sunscreen every day. In some cases, daily use of tretinoin is also recommended and may speed healing. This skin-care regimen will help the skin peel more evenly, will speed healing after the peel, and may reduce the chance of infection and other complications, especially uneven color changes in the skin.

For medium and deep peels of the face, especially in the areas near the mouth or eyes, you may be given a short course of medication (such as acyclovir) a few days before the peel to prevent viral infection.

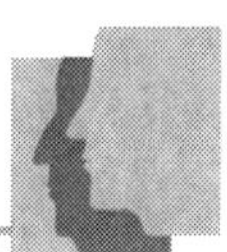

***Procedure***

For a superficial peel, the skin is cleaned immediately before the peel. The chemical (usually a liquid or paste) is then applied to the skin with a small brush, gauze, or cotton-tipped applicators. The chemical is left on the skin for two to seven minutes, depending on the type of chemical used. Water is often used to neutralize the acid and end the chemical reaction, then it is wiped off. You may feel a little burning while the chemical is on your skin. A handheld fan can help cool the skin and relieve any discomfort.

The technique used to do a medium peel is similar to that used for a superficial peel, but the chemical may be left on for a longer period of time. Medium peels are more painful than superficial peels, because the chemicals are stronger and they soak deeper into the skin. You may be given a pain reliever and an oral sedative to reduce pain and anxiety during the procedure. Cool compresses and fans can be used to cool the stinging and burning caused by the chemical. The procedure takes about 20 minutes. There is little or no pain once the peel is finished.

Deep peels take the most time and are the most painful type of chemical peel. The procedure for a deep peel using phenol is also more complicated than for other types of peels:

- You may be given an oral sedative and pain relievers, usually in the form of a shot. General anesthesia is used less often because it increases the risk of complications and is usually not necessary.
- You may be put on a heart monitor and receive IV (intravenous) fluids during the procedure because phenol is toxic when absorbed into the body's systems in large doses. These measures may not be necessary if only a single, small area is being peeled.
- After the skin has been thoroughly cleaned, the chemical will be applied and allowed to penetrate. After one area of the face is treated, there will be a 15-minute break before the next area is treated to avoid getting too much phenol in your system.
- Tape or ointment may sometimes be applied to the area after the

peel to treat deeper problem areas. When tape is used, it is removed after two days. Ointment is washed off with water after 24 hours and then reapplied as needed.

Depending on how large an area is being treated, the entire procedure may take 60 to 90 minutes.

### *Afterwards*

Recovery time after a chemical peel depends on what kind of peel was done and how deep it was. With all types of peels, proper care of the skin after the peel is very important to speed healing, help results last longer, prevent infection, and avoid color changes in the treated area caused by sun exposure. Proper skin care after a peel is similar to the care used to prepare for a peel and typically involves:

- Cleansing the skin frequently with water
- Changing the dressing or ointment on the wound (for medium and deep peels)
- Moisturizing the skin daily
- Avoiding any sun exposure until peeling has stopped and sunscreen can be used

Once peeling has stopped, sunscreen should be used every day. New skin is more susceptible to sun damage. Some doctors may also recommend using tretinoin cream nightly, usually beginning two to three weeks after the peel.

Superficial peels are done on an outpatient basis, do not require anesthesia, and cause only slight discomfort afterwards. Most people can return to their normal activities immediately. The skin heals quickly after a superficial peel. The skin may turn pink, and usually only minimal peeling occurs. You can use makeup to hide any redness until it fades.

Medium peels are usually done on an outpatient basis, but you may need to take a few days off work to recover. A medium peel causes a second-degree burn of the skin. The skin takes five to seven days to heal to a point where you can use makeup to hide the redness

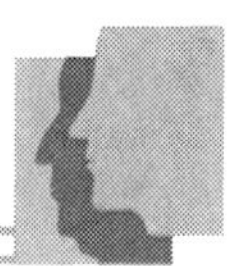

caused by the peel. There is little or no pain after the peel, but there may be some swelling, especially if the area around the eyes is treated. The skin will turn reddish-brown in two to three days, become crusty, and then flake and peel over the next few days.

A deep peel causes a third-degree burn of the skin. Skin regrowth begins within 10 to 14 days after a deep peel, and the skin remains extremely red and tender for up to three weeks. Most people take this time off from work. Complete healing of the skin may take several months.

Oral pain relievers may be given to reduce pain after the peel.

Some people have severe swelling, especially around the eye area. Elevating the head may reduce the swelling to some extent, and corticosteroids may be used for more severe swelling. You may be given a short course of antiviral and antibiotic medications to prevent infection after the peel.

Proper wound care is extremely important after a deep peel to speed healing and prevent infection of the wound. You may be asked to shower several times a day to reduce crusting, and you may have to return to the doctor's office frequently to have the wound cleaned and checked.

### *Contraindications*

A chemical peel (except for a superficial peel) may not be done if you have:

- ♦ Recently used isotretinoin (Accutane, a drug used to treat acne).
- ♦ Had recent facial surgery or facial radiation therapy. This can make regrowth of the skin more difficult.
- ♦ An active herpes infection affecting the area to be treated.
- ♦ An impaired immune system. This can delay healing and increase the risk of infection and skin color changes after the peel.
- ♦ Known allergies to certain medications.

*Results*

The results of a chemical peel depend in part on how deep the peel is. A superficial peel may slightly reduce but does not eliminate sun damage and signs of aging. The results may not appear for some time, and when they do appear, they may be minimal. Repeated peels are often needed to produce the effect the person wants.

A medium peel can be very effective in evening out pigment differences and in reducing fine wrinkles and signs of sun damage. Re-treatment is often needed after three to six months to produce the best effect.

A single deep peel eliminates wrinkles and may tighten the skin. The effects are often dramatic. In general, a person cannot have repeated deep phenol peels.

Your skin type, skin care before and after the peel, the doctor's level of experience, and your lifestyle after the procedure can also affect the results. Some types of skin problems respond better to chemical peeling than others. People with lighter skin who limit their sun exposure after the procedure tend to have better results than those with darker skin and those who continue to spend lots of time in the sun.

Before you decide to have a chemical peel, talk to your doctor about the kind of results you can expect. Changes in the color and texture of the skin caused by aging and sun exposure may continue to develop after a chemical peel. Chemical peels are not a permanent solution for these problems.

*Complications*

In general, the deeper the peel, the greater the risk of side effects and complications. Chemical peels can result in:

♦ Redness (erythema). Expect some redness of the skin after a chemical peel. With deeper peels or with certain skin types, redness can be severe. It may fade within a few weeks, or it may last several months.

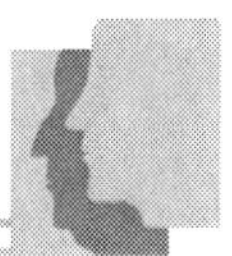

- Color changes in the skin. Treated areas may be darker or lighter than the surrounding skin.
- Crusting and scaling.
- Swelling (edema), especially around the eyes.
- Scarring.
- Allergic reaction to the chemical.
- Infection. People who have a history of herpes outbreaks are especially prone to infection after a chemical peel.
- Increased sensitivity to sunlight.
- Deep peels using phenol can rarely cause more severe complications during the procedure, including heart, liver, or kidney failure.

Chemical peels are designed to wound and remove the upper layers of the skin. You need to prepare yourself for how your skin will look immediately after the peel and throughout the healing process. You also need to be prepared to use cosmetics to blend skin tones between treated and untreated areas, such as between the face and jaw line.

Be sure that your doctor understands what you hope to achieve and that you understand what results you can realistically expect. Even with realistic expectations, you may not see results for several weeks or months after a chemical peel.

During the early healing period after a chemical peel (before the skin has finished peeling), you must avoid sun exposure. Once the early healing period has passed, you will need to wear sunscreen every day and limit sun exposure as much as possible. New skin is more susceptible to damage and discoloration from sunlight.

Chemical peeling, dermabrasion, and laser resurfacing are the most commonly used techniques for improving the texture and appearance of the skin. Although these techniques use different methods, they have basically the same effect on the skin: They destroy and remove the upper layers of skin to allow for skin regrowth.

One technique is not necessarily better than the others. When performed by an experienced surgeon, laser resurfacing may be slightly more precise than chemical peeling or dermabrasion. However, the choice of technique is based on the site you want to treat, your skin type and condition, the doctor's experience, your preferences, and other factors. Some people may get the best results using a combination of techniques, as when chemical peels are coupled with dermabrasion or laser resurfacing for a more dramatic overall effect.

### *New Peeling Techniques*

Recently, two more peeling techniques have become available. The first is the AFA/clay peel, developed by a (of course) California group. AFA stands for "amino acid filaggrin-based antioxidants," which are said to be antioxidants, exfoliants and moisturizers. This technique looks very promising for acne, rosacea and hyperpigmentation. Its main advantage is that it is simple to do and has few side effects.

Vitalaze is a vitamin A acid peel that has the advantage of being very superficial. It is designed for all skin types. Formulated from alpha-hydroxy acids, beta-hydroxy acids, resorcinol, and retinoic acid (obtained by physician) The results are predictable after one peel. After a series, a significant difference is seen.

Also new is ALA/PDT therapy, which we touched on earlier in our discussion of wrinkles In this procedure, a thorough cleansing is done, the ALA agent is applied and then a laser is used to excite it. The main benefit is extreme precision. It appears to offer excellent results for photodamage and acne.

## The Blinking Lights

Recently, a new therapy has been shown to be extremely beneficial for the skin. Unlike chemical peels, which correct damage already done, this therapy maintains healthy skin. The technology is called Gentlewaves®. Treatments are short and average 33 seconds a week.

The uniqueness of this therapy lies in the way it shuts off collagen

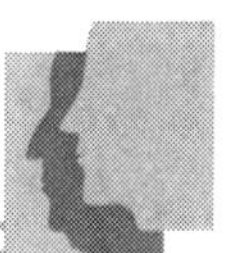

breakdown by inhibiting enzymes that breakdown collagen. It also turns on the microchondria of fibroblast cells. These are the power plant of the cells that produce collagen. As a stand-alone treatment or as a combination with peels or microdermabrasion, Gentlewaves® is proving useful in our quiet war against aging.

## Dermabrasion

*Dermabrasion* removes lines and some scarring and can be used to treat moderate to severe photo (sun) damage. During dermabrasion, the doctor sands away the top layer of skin using a wire brush or diamond wheel. This allows new skin to grow and is most often used to treat acne scars and wrinkles around the mouth. The side effects and complications are similar to those that may follow medium to deep chemical peels: crusting, weeping, oozing and risk of infections that occur because the skins surface has been disrupted.

## Microdermabrasion

Until recently, who knew that a sandstorm could be good for your skin? Yet microdermabrasion is just that: a procedure that blows crystals of aluminum oxide onto the skin and removes them with a vacuum. Statistics say it's currently the most popular cosmetic procedure in the U.S. Both patients and physicians have reported younger looking, smoother skin.

The results of a small study that tested the "sand-blasting" technique reported that six out of 10 of his patients reported mild improvements, and no one was unhappy. But, are the results long lasting? The procedure is too young for us to know.

Microdermabrasion is part of a non-ablative rejuvenation program. At the level of epidermal rejuvenation, these non-ablative options include superficial chemical peeling or this newer procedure. They are used in conjunction with lasers and intense pulse-light sources that target blood vessels and melanin, and lasers that target collagen to rejuvenate all levels of the skin's structures without causing disruption of the epidermis (and without downtime for the patient).

Microdermabrasion is particularly helpful in the early stages of photo-aging and as a program for maintaining the long-term effects of any facial rejuvenation technique. Microdermabrasion also plays a major role in prepping patients for more resurfacing procedures or cosmetic procedures, including deeper chemical peeling. Microdermabrasion has been definitively shown to be helpful in skin resurfacing: to make the skin smoother, improve mild pigmentation problems, reduce pore size, treat acne and pustules and give skin a smoother contour.

Microdermabrasion is most helpful in the treatment of superficial acne scarring associated with inflammatory *acne vulgaris*. The areas where it may have some future applications are in the treatment of scars, stretch marks and other mild disorders of gelatinization, including *keratosis pilaris* and *epidermal melasma*, all described in the section "Acne and Other Skin Ailments."

## Laser Resurfacing

Laser resurfacing uses heat induced by laser light to destroy and remove (vaporize) the upper layers of the skin. This causes new skin to grow. It is typically used to remove or improve the appearance of wrinkles, shallow scars (from acne, surgery, or trauma), tattoos, and other skin defects.

The laser sends out brief pulses of high-energy light that are absorbed by water and certain substances in the skin called chromophores. The light is changed into heat energy, and the heat then vaporizes thin sections of skin, layer by layer. As the wounded area heals, new skin grows to replace the damaged skin that was removed during the laser treatment.

The $CO_2$ (carbon dioxide) laser is the most common type of laser used for resurfacing. Erbium lasers are also used frequently and are growing in popularity because they do a similar job but penetrate less deeply and therefore heal more quickly. Laser resurfacing is

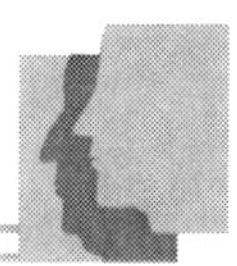

usually very precise and causes little damage to the surrounding skin and tissue. It is done most often on the face, but it may be done on skin in other areas of the body. The hands, neck, and chest are usually avoided because skin in these areas tends to thicken and scar as a result of the laser treatment and does not heal as well as it does in other areas. Some surgeons are willing to treat the neck with a lower-energy laser.

Recently, a whole new generation of lasers has arrived: so-called fractionated resurfacing technology, which we looked at in our section on scarring. Here's how it differs from peels: the laser treats damaged and aging skin by harmlessly penetrating the outer layer of skin, but only resurfacing 15% to 20% of the skin during each session. This method protects the skin from enduring too much damage at once and eliminates much of the downtime associated with $CO_2$ or erbium laser resurfacing treatment. The benefit to you, the patient, is little or no downtime.

The areas to be treated by a resurfacing laser are cleaned and marked with a pen. A nerve block with a local anesthetic is usually used to numb the area before treatment. You may also be given a sedative or anti-anxiety medication such as diazepam (Valium) to help you relax. If your entire face is going to be treated, you may need stronger anesthesia (in some cases, general anesthesia), pain relievers, or sedation. You may be given goggles to wear to prevent eye damage by the laser, and wet towels will be placed around the area to absorb excess laser pulses.

The laser is passed over the skin, sending out pulses. Each pulse lasts less than a millisecond. Between passes with the laser, water or a saline solution is wiped on to cool the skin and remove tissue that the laser has destroyed. The number of passes required depends on how large the area is and what type of skin is being treated. Thin skin around the eyes, for instance, requires very few passes with the laser. Thicker skin or skin with more severe lesions requires a greater number of passes.

The pulses from the laser may sting or burn slightly or you may feel a snapping sensation against your skin. Little or no bleeding occurs in most cases, although severely damaged skin may bleed. When the treatment is finished, the area is covered with a clean dressing or ointment.

Laser resurfacing is usually done in a doctor's office or outpatient surgery center. The time needed for healing and recovery after laser resurfacing varies according to the size and depth of the treated area. Someone who has their full face resurfaced, for example, will require a longer recovery time than someone who has only a small area of skin treated.

In general, the wounded area will be weeping, tender, and swollen for at least several days. Rarely, this can go on for two to three weeks. Cold packs and anti-inflammatory medications (such as acetaminophen or ibuprofen) may help reduce swelling and pain. Once skin regrowth occurs, the skin will remain red for several weeks.

Proper care of the treated area while the skin is healing is extremely important.

- ·Rinse the skin several times a day with cool vinegar-in-water mix to avoid infection and to wash away the crusting that sometimes develops. Avoid soaps and perfumes.
- Change the ointment or dressing on the treated area to keep the area moist and promote healing.
- Avoid sun exposure and, after peeling has stopped, use sunscreen every day. New skin is more susceptible to sun damage.

Your doctor may give you an antiviral drug called acyclovir to prevent infection if a large area of the skin was treated or if you have a history of infection with the herpes simplex virus.

Several follow-up visits to your doctor will be needed to monitor the skin's healing and regrowth and to identify and treat early signs of infection or other complications.

Laser resurfacing may be used to remove or improve the appearance of:

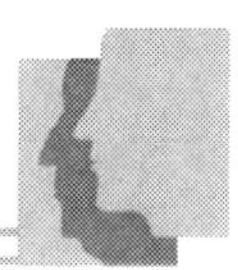

***Wrinkles.***

♦ Superficial scars caused by acne, surgery, or trauma that are not growing or getting thicker.

♦ Color (pigment) changes or defects in the skin, such as liver spots (lentigines), port-wine stains, or coffee spots.

♦ Lesions or growths in the upper layer of skin (such as actinic keratoses, rhinophyma, or birthmarks). Any growth that could be malignant should be evaluated using a biopsy before laser resurfacing is done.

***Tattoos.***

You may not be a good candidate for laser resurfacing if you:

♦ Have had skin color changes, scarring, or thickened tissue (fibrosis) as a result of earlier treatment.

♦ Have a skin, blood flow, or immune disorder that could make healing more difficult.

♦ Have a history of abnormal scarring (keloid or hypertrophic scars).

♦ Are currently using isotretinoin (Accutane, a drug used to treat acne) or have used it within the last six to 12 months. This increases the risk of scarring after the procedure.

♦ Have a bacterial or viral infection of the skin.

Your skin type, the condition of your skin, your doctor's level of experience, the type of laser used, and your lifestyle following the procedure can all affect the short-term and long-term results of laser resurfacing. Some types of skin problems or defects respond better to laser resurfacing than others. People with lighter skin who limit their sun exposure after the procedure tend to have better results than those with darker skin and those who continue to spend lots of time in the sun. People with darker skin may benefit from laser resurfacing, but their skin may not heal as well.

In general, laser resurfacing tends to have good results with fairly low risks. Wrinkles caused by aging and long-term sun exposure, such as those around the eyes and mouth, respond well to laser resurfacing. The long-term results for these types of wrinkles are unknown but I have used this technology for years and have seen very, very few problems. Keep in mind that new wrinkles will probably appear as your skin continues to age. Wrinkles caused by repeated movement and muscle use (such as those on the forehead or along the sides of the nose) may be improved but not eliminated. They often come back months or years after treatment because the muscles continue to perform the activities that caused the wrinkles before treatment.

Mild or moderate acne scars may be somewhat improved. Laser treatment is less effective on severe acne scars.

Side effects and risks of laser resurfacing may include:

♦ Swelling, itching, crusting, and tenderness. These are expected, temporary effects of laser resurfacing.

♦ Redness (erythema). Normally this lasts six to 12 weeks, but it may last up to six months in some people. Some people may turn red or flush during stress or exertion more easily than they used to for up to a year.

♦ Color (pigment) changes in the skin. In 30% to 40% of people, especially those with darker skin tones, the treated skin is darker than the surrounding skin. Bleaching or peeling of the skin can help lighten the skin for a more uniform skin tone, and the skin may fade on its own over time. A small number of people have a loss of color in the treated skin six to 12 months after the procedure. This effect may be permanent, especially with deeper laser treatments.

♦ Skin irritation, including acne flare-ups in people who are prone to acne.

♦ Bacterial, viral, or fungal infection of the skin. Infection may affect the rest of the body as well.

♦ Scarring (rare). Scarring may be improved with medication.

♦ A condition in which the edge of the eyelid rolls outward and exposes the inside of the eyelid (ectropion). This is a rare but

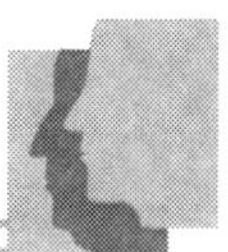

serious complication of laser treatment in the eye area. Surgery is sometimes needed to correct it. It is more likely to occur in people who have a loose lower eyelid or who have had surgery on their lower eyelids (blepharoplasty).

Laser resurfacing wounds and destroys the skin. You need to prepare yourself for how your skin will look immediately after treatment and throughout the healing process. It is also extremely important for you to follow your doctor's instructions on caring for your skin after the treatment to avoid infection and help the skin heal.

Be sure that your doctor understands what you hope to achieve and that you understand what results you can realistically expect. Even with realistic expectations, you may not see results for several weeks or months after laser resurfacing. You may need more than one treatment to achieve the results you want.

After laser resurfacing, you will need to wear sunscreen every day and avoid sun exposure as much as possible. New skin is more susceptible to damage and discoloration from sunlight.

*Non-ablative lasers* that "resurface" without damaging the skin are now replacing resurfacing lasers for some applications. Acne scars, fine lines and even acne are being treated by these innovative machines.

## Thermage and Other Tissue-Tightening Technologies

This is a new, exciting, no-down-time procedure that uses high intensity radio waves, infrared light, or heat to tighten the skin of the face and neck without surgery. It was originally developed by Javier Ruiz-Esparza, a San Diego dermatologist, the first doctor in the world to use this modality for cosmetic purposes and the one with the longest experience in this area.

Thermage and related technologies protect the skin surface with a cooling action while heating the deep layers underneath. The procedure is intended to cause immediate collagen contraction followed by new collagen production and continued tightening over time.

Patients treated in clinical studies continue to show improvement at least six months after treatment. The procedure requires no recovery time, so you can return to normal activities the day after your treatment. Best of all, there are no needles or scalpels, and few reports of damage to the skin surface. Since the Thermage procedure works by tightening the deeper tissue, it can complement other procedures that treat the upper layers of your skin.

I have followed the progress of this technology for several years. After several revisions to the Thermage technology and technique, it has come of age. However, it continues to evolve with better variations still being made. Competing companies with similar technologies are now able to offer good results.

### ALA/PDT

This is a new treatment I've referred to earlier. It employs a photoactive chemical (ALA) that is applied to the skin and then activated by a light source such as a laser or a blue light ("photodynamic therapy" or PDT). This is highly effective in treating photo damage, acne and rosacea.

### Photofacial Rejuvenation

Photo-rejuvenation consists of a series of intense pulsed-light treatments that improve the appearance of rosacea, flushing, broken capillaries, sun-damaged skin, age spots, skin texture and photo-aging. This is not laser light, which is monochromatic (that is, consists of a single wavelength of light) but a broad spectrum of light of many wavelengths. Treatment also improves mild acne scars, reduces large pores, corrects dark circles around the eyes, and reduces fine lines. Treatments are especially effective for improving the appearance of the face, neck, chest, and hands. This exciting treatment involves little or no down time. You can resume normal activities immediately.

An intense light is applied in a series of gentle pulses over the treatment area. Without damaging the skin, the light penetrates

through the skin and is absorbed by the abnormally dilated vessels or pigmentation. The heat causes damage to the vessel or lesion, and the body begins its natural healing process. The lesion will darken before it flakes off or the body absorbs it. Treatment can be given as frequently as every three weeks.

For optimal results, a series of three to five treatments are recommended. You may decide to have follow-up treatments once a year to maintain results. Treatment may vary from 15 to 45 minutes depending on the size of the area to be treated. We first cleanse the area to be treated and apply a cool gel. When the pulse of light is delivered, the patient experiences a sensation similar to the snap of a rubber band. After treatment, we remove the gel, cleanse the skin and apply a sunscreen. Pain is minimal, though a topical anesthesia provides maximum comfort. For sensitive skin, we apply a cool compress following treatment.

Side effects are rare. Immediately following treatment, the skin may appear flushed, brown pigmented spots may appear darker, and capillaries may be more visible. In rare instances, temporary swelling and/or blistering can occur.

Patients have a high degree of satisfaction with their results. Expect to see a gradual decrease in redness, broken capillaries, flushing, irregular pigmentation, pore size and fine lines. After each treatment, the skin will feel smoother and appear to have a more even tone.

## Fillers

If you have thin lips or deep creases anywhere on your face or neck, there are many exciting advances in cosmetic surgery to help you. Known as "fillers," they fill in wrinkles and depressed scars and many different filler options have come to the forefront over the last few years.

The first of these was collagen. Its utility was limited by three factors. First, some people were allergic to it so pre-testing was necessary in all patients. Second, when injected, it didn't last long. Third, because this product was made from bovine sources, the recent epidemic of mad cow disease in Europe and Canada has rendered this product less than ideal.

Fortunately, the industry has responded with a plethora of options. In fact, in Europe, which is the acknowledged leader in this area, there are over 70 different options.

Amongst the most popular of these are what are known as NASHA (for "non-animal stabilized hyaluronic acid") products. The first of these was made by Medics Corp. of Sweden. It is called Restylane and is available in Canada and the United States. Since being introduced it has given birth to a whole new family of products including Perlane, a thicker product for deeper lines, and Restylane, a thinner product for finer lines.

As I wrote earlier, these products are made of hyaluronic acid (HA), a material naturally found in the dermis of the skin. Because natural HA wouldn't last long (the body has enzymes that degrade it), Medicis has made a stabilized variety that degrades slowly, and when it degrades, it traps more water, maintaining its correction for an average of nine months in most patients.

I love this material. It's like painting with water colors and a fine paint brush. In most patients results are predictable and long lasting, making treatments easy. No need to live with the ugly unwanted lines of aging any longer.

Recently, a competitor has entered the scene with another NASHA product: Juvederm®. It's too early to tell whether it will be as good.

For those who are looking for even longer-lasting results, a group of super long lasting products have come on the market. These are Radiesse, Artefill, Artecoll and Sculptra. Artefill and Artecoll are combinations of collagen and PMMA, a material more commonly known as Plexiglass. When this combination is put into the body, the collagen is rapidly degraded leaving the PMMA behind. The body walls of the PMMA leave a long lasting correction. How long? Some reports suggest as long as 20 years.

No doubt many more products will enter this field. Recently, Sculptura® has been introduced in the U.S. and Canada. It lasts three years and acts as a "stimulatory filler" literally stimulating the body to produce collagen. Several other long lasting fillers are also recently available. There are now many options for doctor and patient—and options are nothing but good.

## Botox

Botox is the most popular cosmetic procedure in the world. It's quick, comparatively cheap and in vogue. You've probably heard about the Hollywood Botox parties. But is it safe?

Botulinum toxin (Botox, for short) is produced by the bacteria *clostridium botulinum*. When this toxin is injected into a muscle, it blocks nerve signals that tell the muscle to contract. This temporarily weakens or paralyzes the muscle and has the effect of smoothing or eliminating wrinkles in the skin. Getting a Botox injection takes just a few minutes. You can return to your regular activities immediately after the injection. The effects of the injection on the targeted areas are usually immediate, though they may take three to four days to appear in some cases. The results may last for up to 120 days. After that you will begin to see the wrinkles return.

Botox injections are used to reduce facial wrinkles in motion. Botulinum toxin has also been used to treat eye muscle disorders, including strabismus, and abnormal neck and shoulder contractions.

Is Botox safe? There are certainly side effects, the most common being headache, bruising, flu-like symptoms, drooping eyelid (ptosis) and nausea. Other side effects include temporary facial pain, redness at the injection site, and weakness in the muscles of the face. In extreme cases, this muscle weakness can limit your facial expressions.

The long-term effects of repeated Botox injections are not known.

Botox injections are more convenient and less painful than other procedures—chemical peels, dermabrasion, laser resurfacing, facelift—that reduce wrinkles and make your face look younger. But since the effects of an injection last only a few months, to maintain the effects, you will have to receive injections a few times per year. While a single injection may seem inexpensive, the cost of repeated injections can quickly add up.

***Botox Safety***

Botox is available only by prescription and must only be used under strict medical supervision. Botox was first approved in 1989 to treat eye-muscle disorders and in 2000 to treat a nerve disorder called cervical dystonia, which causes severe neck and shoulder contractions. In April 15, 2002, the FDA approved the use of Botox injections in the U.S.A. to temporarily reduce the appearance of frown lines and wrinkles between the eyebrows. It is also approved for this indication in Canada. The product had already been widely used for this purpose by dermatologists, plastic surgeons and other doctors, but official approval gives the manufacturer formal permission to market it as a wrinkle reducer.

The FDA based its approval for this new use of Botox on several clinical trials involving a total of 405 people with moderate-to-severe frown lines between the eyebrows (known as glabellar lines). Test subjects were injected with Botox or a placebo. After 30 days, the great majority of researchers and patients observed the frown lines to be improved or nonexistent. Very few people in the placebo group saw similar results.

The appearance of these frown lines was reduced for up to 120 days in the Botox group. It's recommended that the drug be used no more frequently than once every three months and at the lowest possible dose.

Still, the question remains: Is Botox too good to be true?

In a 2003 issue of the *AMA Journal*, one expert wonders whether we really know the potential long-term effects of this wrinkle-smoothing drug.

When injected in small doses into specific muscles, the toxin

smoothes wrinkles by paralyzing those muscles. Though the FDA has approved Botox only for wrinkles between the eyebrows, the toxin is commonly used cosmetically in other areas, such as the forehead and around the eyes.

Botox is still a key ingredient in biochemical warfare, and there are reports that Saddam Hussein's Iraq "favored" this toxin over anthrax and other poisons. But research suggests the same effect that makes it so effective in weapons of mass destruction provides for some darn versatile medicine. Recent studies indicate that Botox's muscle-relaxing action appears effective in treating a host of conditions including bladder dysfunction, excessive sweating, cerebral palsy, post-stroke spasticity, back pain, and even anal fissures.

Some of the most promising research, however, has been in using this "wrinkle remedy" as a treatment for headaches. In June, findings of 13 studies presented at the American Headache Society annual meeting suggested that Botox was effective in reducing migraines and other severe headaches. The underlying mechanism isn't clear, but some researchers believe Botox blocks nerves that relay pain messages to the brain and relaxes muscles, making them less sensitive to pain.

In Canada, Botox has been a welcomed addition to the cosmetic regimen and is a cornerstone of treating cosmetic problems. It is often used with fillers, IPLs, lifters, cosmetic products and Thermage®. Botox injections usually range from about $300 to $2000 per treatment but may be higher in certain areas of the country.

One last word of caution. Recently, a Florida chiropractor injected not-for-human-use botulism toxin into some patients, resulting in paralysis of the body. Beware. Choose your Botox doctor carefully.

## Sclerotherapy

Sclerotherapy is a procedure for the treatment of small varicose veins and spider veins. A chemical is injected into a vein to damage and scar the interior lining of the vein, which causes the vein to close.

Lasers are also used sometimes to treat small veins.

### "Antiptosis" or "Aptos" or "Russian" Thread

The hallmark of the aging face is falling features. Jowls begin to develop, the forehead droops producing baggy upper lids, the neck sags and smile lines become dramatically more noticeable. The causes of these changes are the normal aging process coupled with the individual's genetic code. Everyone is affected to some degree. I always tell my patients: "That's why you should choose your parents wisely."

As we've seen, a physician's armamentarium of techniques to diminish the effect of these changes consisted until recently of the surgical face-lift (the S-lift, the lifting of the superficial musculoaponeurotic system (SMAS), the traditional face-lift, the mini-lift, etc.), laser treatments ($CO_2$, Erbium, and IPL), chemical peels (phenol, TCA, Baker-Gordon, Jessner's), dermabrasion, and medicated cream programs. Their main problem was this: concomitant to the degree of improvement was the degree of difficulty and complications. Yes, we *could* get great results, but with significant risk and downtime.

However, a new technology—"Russian thread," also known as the Aptos (for "*a*nti-*ptos*is," ptosis originally referring to the sagging of the eyelid) Intradermal Suspension Thread—has now been added to these other tools.

The first development of anything like intradermal threads to correct and/or prevent facial ptosis took place in the 1970s, when the superficial musculoaponeurotic system (SMAS), part of the anatomy of the cheek, was described by Mitz and Peironye and led to more sophisticated lifting procedures to off-set the effects of gravity.

In 1999, Russian scientist, inventor, and cosmetic surgeon Dr. Marlen Sulamanidze, along with his son, Dr. Georges Sulamanidze and with Dr. Tatiana Paikidze, re-invented and improved this non-surgical facial rejuvenation method.

Since then, many variations of the procedure have occurred. Surgeons insert threads measuring from 5 cm to 18 cm in length and the

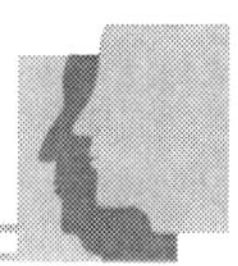

patterns of insertion vary widely. These have recently evolved into the state-of-the-art Silhouette thread from KMI.

These threads are specially designed barbed polypropylene #2-0 and #3-0 strings that attach to and strongly anchor to the dermis, lifting and suspending the skin and subcutaneous fat in the process. The result is a visible yet subtle facial rejuvenation.

In many ways, the threading procedure is superior to other face-lifting procedures. The major benefits to the patient over the procedures that have been available include the following:

- ♦ No major trauma. Most patients can return to work immediately or within a few days.
- ♦ No major scars. The threads are always inserted through puncture wounds that heal virtually invisibly.
- ♦ Low risk compared to existing procedures.
- ♦ The technique is relatively easy to learn and perform.
- ♦ No general or tumescent anesthesia is necessary, allowing for a rapid recovery.
- ♦ The procedure is quick. Most cases take less than an hour to do.
- ♦ The procedure is virtually bloodless and painless.
- ♦ There is little pain and swelling following the procedure.

Russian thread procedures successfully reverse the sagging process that occurs as a result of aging, and does so quickly, effectively, and with minimal downtime. It is a revolutionary breakthrough. I was one of the first physicians in North America to offer it, having studied the technique in Mexico with Dr. Carl Bazan, of Aguascalientes. Dr. Bazan is a world expert in the technique.

The best candidates for this procedure are those younger patients who do not have redundant skin. Patients with more redundancy of the skin would probably be best treated by other modalities, such as $CO_2$ resurfacing, or a more traditional face-lifting procedure.

The thread procedure appears to be effective with:

- ♦ removal of "crow's feet"
- ♦ forehead lift

- cheek lift, cheek augmentation or rejuvenation
- smile lines
- nasolacrimal folds
- nasolabial folds
- mid-face sagging
- jowls and the loss of mandibular rim definition
- neck rejuvenation.

I would never perform this procedure on patients with severe health problems. And there are also certain circumstances under which I would not recommend this procedure:

- unrealistic expectations in the patient
- illegal medication or substance abuse
- severe systemic illness
- local or systemic infection
- anti-coagulation.

I would be extremely cautious if my patient smoked, had a history of facial and scalp eczema or psoriasis, or a history of keloidal or hypertrophic scarring.

The procedure takes about one hour to an hour and a half. That's why we call it the "lunchtime facelift"—you can have it done at lunchtime. And although the Russian thread is a relatively new procedure, the response has been amazing. A patient, Judy K., a 57-year-old secretary, wrote to say:

> I used to love the way I looked, but when I hit the big 5-0, things began to change—and not necessarily for the better! My jowls really began to show "those changes." Yucky laugh lines began to show. I thought I needed a facelift, but I didn't want the downtime associated with it.
>
> The Contour thread has changed my life forever! The most amazing thing. I had it done and was back at work the next day. Yes, I had a bit of bruising. But, wow…in three weeks I looked great!

Recently, the Canadian distributor has ceased the sale of the older

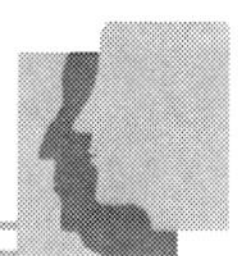

thread product for unknown reasons. The Silhouette thread is expected to replace it shortly.

### Lipoplasty

Sometimes called body sculpting, lipoplasty removes stubborn pockets of fat such as "saddle bags" and "love handles" that don't conform to a person's ideal body image. The surgeon simply vacuums out the fat through a small incision. We're going to have a detailed look at the procedure in our chapter on the body.

Many people are unaware that liposuction can also be employed on problem areas such as the neck, the area just below the bra and even the "banana roll" area between the buttock and the back of the thigh.

### Mesotherapy

Mesotherapy is a new way to dissolve fat through a series of injections. It is a simpler, less invasive technique than liposuction. Mesotherapy is sometimes used to treat fat under the eyes, but because, like liposuction, it finds most of its applications below the neck, we'll discuss it in detail in our chapter on the body. A refinement of mesotherapy known as "lipodissolve" has recently come into vogue and brought improved results.

### Laser Lipolysis

Recently, Cynosure Lasers has released the "Smart Laser" to be used alone or in combination with liposuction. The benefits are that it melts the fat before suctioning is done, thus decreasing trauma and helping to contract loose skin. The end result for the patient is less downtime and improved results. Meanwhile, Meridian lasers has produced a low-light laser that can remove fat without any trauma or surgery. Although new, we have found patients lose several inches with several treatment sessions by a Meridian laser.

## Caring for Your Face: "Aggressive" Cosmetic Surgery

Much like the cosmetic procedures I've described above, more aggressive cosmetic surgery is done to change some aspect of a person's appearance or function. It is often considered elective surgery—that is, not necessary for medical reasons—but there sometimes *are* medical and functional reasons for having cosmetic surgery: some medical conditions cause problems that may be improved or repaired by cosmetic surgery.

Cosmetic surgery includes reconstructive and non-reconstructive procedures.

*Reconstructive surgery.* A person who seeks reconstructive surgery typically has a noticeable disfigurement (such as a scar, skin condition, or malformed body part) caused by injury, disease, or birth defect, and this disfigurement makes a strong impact on his or her day-to-day life, affecting social, employment and recreational opportunities as well as self-esteem.

*Non-reconstructive surgery.* A person who seeks non-reconstructive cosmetic surgery is usually unhappy with some aspect of his or her appearance, such as a big nose, small breasts, wrinkles, or "love handles." These kinds of flaws don't bother everyone who has them—some people wouldn't consider them flaws at all—but they can affect the self-image and confidence of others. Cosmetic surgery is one way to address this problem.

This section is primarily about non-reconstructive surgery, though some of the issues discussed may be relevant to reconstructive surgery as well.

So-called aggressive surgery is most often performed under general anesthesia and it usually requires several weeks or even months before the final results can be seen. The length of time for recovery varies greatly depending on the extent of surgery and the general physical condition of the patient.

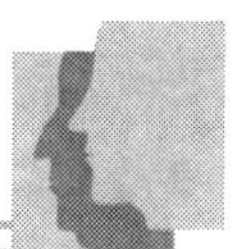

## Eyelid Surgery

*Eyelid surgery* (called *blepharoplasty*) reshapes eyelids to remove bagginess and tighten lose skin around the eyelids, but doesn't remove fine wrinkle lines. Patients experience some swelling and bruising afterward and sometimes the swelling doesn't go down for a week or two. The bruises usually go away in a week to 10 days. Vision may be blurry for days after the operation, and patients may experience dry eyes or may tear up easily. Costs start around $2,000 but can exceed $4,000 depending on the surgeon and the amount of reshaping needed.

## Rhinoplasty

Rhinoplasty is surgery to reshape the nose and can change the size, shape, and angle of the nose to bring it into better proportion with the rest of the face. It can alter the tip of the nose, correct bumps, indentations or other defects. Rhinoplasty may also correct structural problems with the nose that may be causing chronic congestion and breathing problems.

Surgeons who perform rhinoplasties typically have training in plastic surgery, otorhinolaryngology (the ear, nose, and throat specialty) or both.

During rhinoplasty, the surgeon makes incisions to access the bones and cartilage that support the nose. The incisions are usually made inside the nose so that they are invisible after the surgery. Depending on the desired result, some bone and cartilage may be removed, or tissue may be added, either a synthetic filler or tissue from another part of the body. After the surgeon has rearranged and reshaped the bone and cartilage, the skin and tissue is redraped over the structure of the nose. A splint is placed outside the nose to support the new shape of the nose as it heals. Nasal packing may be used inside the nose to provide additional support.

Rhinoplasty may be done using general or local anesthesia. It is often done as an outpatient procedure but sometimes requires a one-night stay in the hospital or surgery center.

If you undergo a rhinoplasty, any surgical packing inside your nose will be removed within a few days after surgery. The doctor will remove the splint and bandaging around your nose after about a week. Your face will feel puffy and the area around your eyes and nose will be bruised and swollen for several days. Cold compresses can help minimize the swelling and reduce pain. Your doctor may also recommend pain medication.

You may need to keep your head elevated and relatively still for the first few days after surgery and it may be several weeks before you can return to strenuous activities.

The results of rhinoplasty may be minor or significant, depending on what kind of correction you want. It is important that you and your plastic surgeon agree on the goals of the surgery. If your expectations are realistic and your plastic surgeon shares them, he or she will probably be able to give you the results you want.

The results of rhinoplasty are permanent, although subsequent injury or other factors can alter the nose's appearance. Cosmetic surgery should only be done on a fully developed nose; complete development has usually occurred by age 15 or 16 in females and by age 17 or 18 in males. If surgery is done before this time, continued development of the nose can alter the surgical results and possibly cause complications.

You can expect temporary swelling and bruising around the eyes and nose after rhinoplasty. Other problems that may occur include:

- bleeding
- skin problems, including breakdown of skin tissue (skin necrosis) and irritation from the tape and bandaging
- infection (Preventive antibiotics may be given after surgery to reduce the risk of infection.)
- serious nasal blockage caused by swelling inside the nose
- complications of anesthesia.

It is also possible that the cosmetic results of the surgery will not be those you wanted.

One of the prominent features of the face, the nose can have a big impact on your self-image and appearance. If you're unhappy with your nose and have been so for a long time, rhinoplasty is a reasonable option to consider. As with other cosmetic procedures, you are more likely to be happy with the results of rhinoplasty if you have clear, realistic expectations about what the surgery can achieve and you share these with your plastic surgeon.

Most insurance companies (and Canadian medicare) will not cover the costs of rhinoplasty unless it is being done to correct a functional problem or a defect caused by disease or injury. Even in these cases, be sure to check with your insurance company to find out what portion of the costs it will cover. Costs of surgery include not only the surgeon's fee but also fees for the operating facility, the anesthesiologist, medications, splints, and packing and other services and materials.

The current cost of a rhinoplasty surgery is around $6,000 and varies by surgeon and location.

## The Facelift

The skin of your face tends to sag and fold as you age. A facelift stretches the skin up toward the scalp, tightening and smoothing it. After the surgery, you will have swelling and bruising. The bruising fades in about two weeks but the swelling may last longer. You may also have some numbness in your face, which can last several weeks. You should be able to get back into your normal routine about two weeks after the operation. During the first few days of recovery, you shouldn't do much at all except stay out of the sun. A facelift costs upwards from $5,000.

A facelift is perhaps the most famous and definitely the most comprehensive approach to treating the wrinkles and sagging of the face caused by age. The skin is literally lifted off the face so that the structures beneath the skin can be tightened and the skin can be smoothed over the face.

During the procedure, the surgeon makes an incision that starts in the temple area and circles the ear. The skin is raised, and the muscle and tissue underneath is tightened. The surgeon may remove some fat and skin. The skin is then redraped over the face and sutured. The incision usually falls along the hairline or in a place where the skin would naturally crease so that it does not show after the surgery.

The surgery usually takes several hours. You may be able to go home that day, but people sometimes spend one night in the hospital. Your face will be bandaged after the surgery. The dressings are usually removed one to two days later. If a drainage tube has been placed (usually behind your ear), it will also be removed one to two days after the surgery. Your doctor will remove your stitches within five to 10 days.

Most people have very little pain after the surgery, but your doctor may prescribe pain medication for you in case you do have pain. Swelling and bruising of the face always occur; cold compresses can help relieve these side effects. Your doctor may instruct you to keep your head elevated and still as much as possible. It is also important to avoid smoking for two to four weeks before and after surgery. Smoking increases the risk for skin and tissue death and will delay your face's healing process.

Most people can return to their normal activities two to three weeks after a facelift. At first your face will feel stiff and probably look and feel strange to you. This is normal, but it is important to be prepared for it. Numbness of the skin may last for weeks or months after the surgery. Your skin may feel rough and dry for a few months. Men sometimes have to shave in new places because the skin has been rearranged, but the surgeon can sometimes avoid this.

Facelifts are done to make an older face look younger by eliminating wrinkles and tightening the skin. Having a facelift can make your face appear younger and healthier. Your face will continue to age, but a facelift does indeed "take years off" your face. For some people this may increase self-confidence and reduce anxiety over growing older.

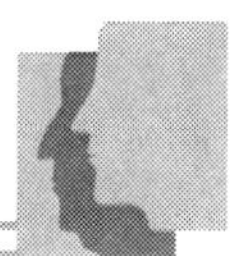

Problems that may be caused by having a facelift include:

- ♦ hair loss (alopecia)
- ♦ bleeding under the skin
- ♦ damage to the nerves that supply the muscles of the face (This can cause paralysis or spasm in the face, but the effects are usually temporary.)
- ♦ infection
- ♦ reactions to the anesthesia.

As with all cosmetic procedures, there is also the risk that the results will not be what you expected. However, an experienced plastic surgeon can usually give you a very clear idea of what to expect after surgery.

As with other cosmetic procedures, you are more likely to be happy with the results of your facelift if you have clear, realistic expectations about what the surgery can achieve and you share these expectations with your plastic surgeon.

Insurance companies do not cover the costs of facelifts. Make sure you know what the total costs of the procedure will be. Costs of surgery include not only the surgeon's fee but also fees for the operating facility, the anesthesiologist, medications, office visits, and other services and materials.

## The "Weekend Alternative to the Facelift"

Dermatologists and surgeons around the world are developing new technologies that will deliver better cosmetic services. With the current focus on minimally invasive procedures, one revolutionary cosmetic surgery technique caught the attention of doctors and the media.

This procedure, called the "weekend alternative to the facelift," available exclusively at one California medical center where it was rapidly gaining popularity, was performed under local anesthesia and was being heralded by some as the future of cosmetic surgery.

The procedure was developed by the cosmetic surgery

husband-and-wife team of William R. Cook Jr., MD, and Kim K. Cook, MD, of Laser Cosmetic Skin Rejuvenation at the Coronado Skin Medical Center Inc., in Coronado, California. The Weekend Alternative to the Facelift was becoming known as a safe and fast alternative to the traditional facelift.

The procedure is performed under local anesthesia, so it should be safer than procedures done under general anesthesia. The surgeon makes a small, hidden incision in the natural fold under the chin. Then, instead of using a scalpel, the surgeon uses a laser, liposuction, and sometimes a chin implant to eliminate the appearance of a sagging face, jowls, and neck.

Unlike conventional facelift surgery, which can leave patients with undesirable scars and a pulled, unnatural appearance, the results of the new technique were said to give more natural appearance with virtually no pain. After a short recovery, the patient could return to normal activity, the only evidence that the procedure has been performed being a dramatically improved appearance and a one-inch incision hidden in the natural fold under the chin. The procedure looked impressive and showed great results without the scars of a traditional facelift surgery. The only downside seemed to be that its use was pretty much limited to the lower face.

In 2004, Dr. William Cook's license was suspended by the California Board of Physicians on the grounds that he "committed acts constituting gross negligence, incompetence, repeated negligent acts, acts of dishonesty, aided the unlicensed practice of medicine, and failed to maintain adequate and accurate records in his care and treatment of four patients." This brought the "weekend alternative to the facelift" into immediate disrepute. It is too early to tell whether this technique will resurface in another form, as many procedures do.

# Chapter 4

# Your Body

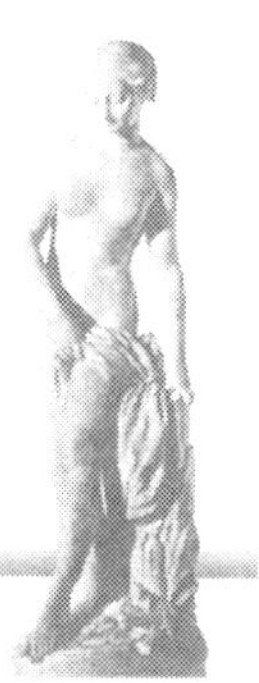

## Cosmetic Surgery and Your Body

Your body is an important part of how you view yourself and an integral part of how you project yourself to the world. Think for a moment about common sayings. How do you feel when someone says a man has a "beer belly" or "love handles"? And what is it that makes beautiful actresses beautiful? Many equate this with an "hour glass" figure.

It may surprise you to know that many cosmetic surgeons think of cosmetic procedures as "above the neck" and "below the neck." This is because these areas heal differently and, as a result, surgeons must employ different cosmetic procedures in these different areas.

You may also have noticed that many people find it easier to retain a youthful body than a youthful face. That's because the sun has such an impact on our facial features, as well as our emotions.

## Caring for Your Body: Cosmetic Procedures

### Liposuction

This procedure is the dream of many men and women battling a cosmetic weight problem or stubborn excess fat. Liposuction is the removal of that fat from the body using a suction apparatus and cannules—small, thin, blunt-tipped tubes. In traditional liposuction, the cannules are inserted through tiny incisions in the skin. Fat is suctioned out through the cannulas as the doctor moves the cannula around under the skin to target specific fat deposits.

In recent years, doctors who perform liposuction have improved on the traditional technique to make it safer, easier, and less painful. Hence, it is often referred to as liposculpture or body sculpturing. These newer techniques include:

♦ **Tumescent liposuction.** This is considered the safest and most effective liposuction technique, with the quickest recovery time. In tumescent liposuction, a large amount of an anesthetic solution containing lidocaine and epinephrine is injected into the fatty tissue before traditional liposuction is performed. The solution makes the fat expand and become firmer, which allows the cannula to move more smoothly under the skin. It also causes the blood vessels to shrink temporarily (vasoconstriction), which greatly reduces blood loss during the procedure. With the large volume of anesthetic solution injected, tumescent liposuction rarely requires general anesthesia (which makes you sleep through the procedure) and thus does not carry some of the risks of traditional liposuction. It also reduces the bruising, swelling and pain that follow the procedure.

♦ **Ultrasound-assisted (ultrasonic) liposuction.** This newer technique uses energy generated by ultrasound to liquefy the fat before it is removed. It actually consists of two types of procedures: intrinsic and extrinsic. In extrinsic liposuction, an ultrasound machine is used outside the body, similar to that used by physiotherapists. In intrinsic liposuction, ultrasound is used to heat the cannula that removes the fat. The benefit is that the cannula moves more smoothly under the skin once the fat has been liquefied, so this technique may be particularly helpful in areas where the fat is very firm or fibrous (such as the sides, the back, male breasts, and the area around the navel). It may also be used when removing large amounts of fat. However the safety of intrinsic ultrasonic liposuction has not been established and this form of ultrasound-assisted liposuction may take two to four hours longer than traditional or tumescent liposuction.

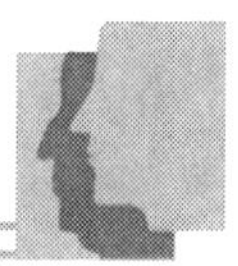

♦ **Power Assisted Liposuction.** Powered instruments allow small cannulas to be used, resulting in less trauma for the patient.

♦ **Laser Assisted Liposuction**. In the autumn of 2006, Cynosure introduced laser liposuction, also called laser lipolysis or "Smart-Lipo." It's been around Europe, Asia, and South America for a few years, and last November, the FDA gave the SmartLipo machine the thumbs up for use in the U.S. It's been recently approved in Canada as well. A recent *People* article reported that, "Smart Lipo may be as close as humans can come to that fat-melting fantasy." It has the added advantage of contracting skin.

Liposuction is usually done as an outpatient procedure in a properly equipped doctor's office, ambulatory surgery center or hospital. In general it does not require an overnight hospital stay unless a large volume of fat is being removed. Local anesthesia is used in most cases and you may or may not be given a sedative to help relax. If traditional (non-tumescent) liposuction is being done, or if a large area or volume of fat is being treated, general anesthesia or deep sedation with an intravenous anesthetic may be used.

After the procedure, the area of the body that was treated is tightly wrapped to help reduce swelling, bruising, and pain. Elastic bandages and tape, support hose (such as those used to treat varicose veins), a special girdle, or another type of tight-fitting garment may be used, depending on which part of the body was treated. You may have to wear the compression garment or wrap for a month or more.

If you have had tumescent liposuction, fluid may drain from the incision sites for several days. In some cases, you may be given antibiotics to reduce the risk of infection.

Most people are able to get up and move around as soon as the treatment is finished and the effects of the anesthesia and any sedation have worn off. You can return to normal activities as soon as it feels comfortable to do so. Many people can return to work within a few days, though this may take as long as a few weeks. Recovery may take longer if you have large areas treated.

The main purpose of liposuction is to reshape an area (or areas) of the body, not to reduce body weight. Liposuction is typically used on "problem" areas that do not respond well to diet and exercise, such as the outer thighs and hips on women ("saddlebags") and the waist and back on men ("love handles"). The face, neck, abdomen, back, buttocks, legs, and upper arms are all commonly treated areas. It is sometimes used in combination with other cosmetic surgery procedures, such as a tummy tuck (abdominoplasty), breast reduction, or facelift.

Liposuction may also be used to treat certain medical conditions, including:

- ♦ Benign fatty tumors (lipomas).
- ♦ Abnormal enlargement of the male breasts (gynecomastia or pseudogynecomastia).
- ♦ Problems with metabolism of fat in the body (lipodystrophy).
- ♦ Excessive sweating in the armpit area (axillary hyperhidrosis).

Liposuction is usually very effective at removing fat deposits in small areas. Some improvement in body contour is usually noticeable right after surgery, but improvement may continue for several weeks (or even months) as the swelling goes away. The full effects of having liposuction may not be visible for several months to a year.

Liposuction does not always tighten the skin over the treated area. After fat has been removed, the skin around the area may be somewhat loose, though in many cases it retracts. It may take up to six months for the skin to tighten around the treated area. Some people's skin is very elastic and retracts more quickly; other people's skin may not tighten up as quickly or as completely. Younger skin tends to have greater elasticity than older skin.

Liposuction done by an experienced doctor in a properly equipped facility is usually safe. Having too many areas treated, or having a very large area treated, may increase the risk of complications during or after the procedure. Tumescent liposuction is considered the safest technique. Side effects may include:

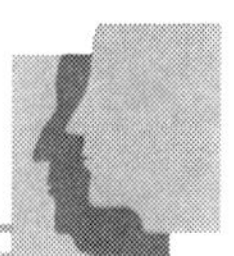

- Temporary swelling, bruising, soreness, and numbness in and around the treated areas. (Tumescent liposuction minimizes these effects in comparison to traditional liposuction.)
- Irritation and minor scarring around the incision sites where the cannulas were inserted.
- Baggy or rippling skin. The skin will usually tighten and retract after a few months. In some people, however, the skin may remain somewhat loose.

Other complications are not common, but they may include:

- Permanent color changes in the skin.
- Uneven skin surface over the treated area.
- Infection. In some cases, antibiotics may be given before or after liposuction to help prevent infection.
- Damage to the nerves and skin. The heat generated during ultrasonic liposuction may burn the skin or damage the tissue under the skin.
- Excessive blood and fluid loss, leading to shock. This is extremely unlikely with the tumescent and ultrasonic techniques, because they usually result in very little blood loss.
- Fat clots or blood clots, which may travel to the lungs (pulmonary embolism) and become life-threatening. (Almost unheard of with tumescent liposuction.)
- Allergic reaction to the injected solution (lidocaine toxicity).

Liposuction is not used to treat obesity and it will not get rid of cellulite or stretch marks. People who expect liposuction to help them lose weight are usually disappointed. Liposuction is not a substitute for exercise and a balanced diet if you are trying to lose weight. In fact, most cosmetic surgeons agree that the best candidates for liposuction are healthy people who are at or close to a healthy weight but who have stubborn fat deposits that do not respond to exercise. However, I have treated less than desirable candidates with pleasing results. The results of liposuction can be long-lasting if you exercise regularly, eat a balanced diet, and maintain a healthy weight after the procedure. When people gain weight after having liposuction, the fatty bulges that were removed often return.

In response to the negative reports in the press, over the last few years the American Society of Aesthetic Plastic Surgeons (ASAPS) sought to determine the main factors increasing the risks associated with liposuction. They found that poor patient health, excessive fat removal, using too much intravenous fluid, general anesthesia during the procedure, and performing multiple procedures during the same surgical session are the factors that are most likely to increase the risk of a patient dying. The ASAPS then launched an education campaign to alert plastic surgeons to the liposuction risk factors and to guide them in the selection of appropriate candidates for the procedure. The findings released from the latest study suggest that this campaign was effective: 94,000 people underwent liposuction by board certified plastic surgeons from September 1998 to September 2000. No major incidents were reported during that period.

Overall, the risks were highest when liposuction was combined with other procedures. For example, when liposuction is performed with a surgical procedure called an abdominoplasty, or "tummy tuck," the rate of deaths was 14 times higher than when lipoplasty was performed alone. Other risk factors include excessive removal of fat and operating on someone in poor health. The new results suggest that fewer surgeons are doing large-volume liposuction and 98.4% of plastic surgeons said they would deny the procedure to people with a serious medical problem.

These new findings translate to a remarkable safety record. The rarity of significant complications means that patients can have a sense of security about elective cosmetic surgery. One of the problems with liposuction is that it can be performed in their office by surgeons, non-surgeons and people with no credentials whatsoever. Personally, I believe you should choose your cosmetic doctor wisely. When it comes to liposuction, we are dealing with a service, not a product. Legitimate doctors caution against going to a doctor who

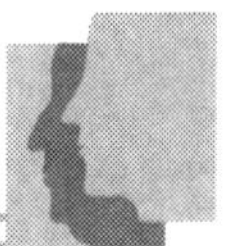

has had a weekend course in liposuction—and yes, that can happen. People interested in liposuction should go to a physician recommended by the Ethical Cosmetic Surgery Association (www.ecsa-online.com).

Meanwhile, many advanced and experienced surgeons are using new techniques to make the procedure even less dangerous and invasive. A new type of liposuction device, for example, may make getting the body-shaping procedure a considerably less serious undertaking. The established manual approach requires the physician to push the tube into the patient, up to ten inches at a time, breaking up fatty deposits and then extracting them with a vacuum pump—a painful and exhausting process for both patients and doctors. This power-assisted liposuction, which employs a power-assisted cannula that moves back and forth up to 5,000 times a minute, can now suck out fat while the patient actually enjoys it, is far more precise than the manual technique, and is considered particularly valuable in difficult-to-reach areas, including the breasts, inner thighs, and around the bellybutton. The FDA approved this device about two years ago, and it has been used successfully on tens of thousands of patients. The power-boosted cannula removes 30% more fat than the traditional manual one. In addition, 54% of patients who underwent powered liposuction on one side of their body and manual liposuction on the other side said they preferred the newer approach; 46% had no preference, and no one said he would rather have the manual technique. Costs range anywhere from $5,000 to $25,000 for the procedure.

### Mesotherapy and Lipodissolve

The battle against fat and cellulite is not won but the weapons are changing. Recently, surgeons have been using a new cosmetic technique to tackle upper arms that flap, inner thighs that jiggle and those love handles that no one loves. Instead of going under the knife, a growing number of patients are tackling fat with a series of injections. The procedure is called mesotherapy and it is taking North

America by storm.

When my friend Dr. Tony Lockwood, a plastic surgeon in Winnipeg, introduced me to this procedure, my first reaction was "Wow!" followed by healthy skepticism. But within a few months, I became an advocate for a procedure that really works

Mesotherapy is growing in popularity because it is a simpler, less invasive technique than liposuction. The abdomen, especially the upper abdomen, the flanks, the neck, bulging lower eyelids, the inner thighs, the knees, the saddlebags and the inferior buttocks are the best areas for treatment, though other areas such as the arms, the jowls, and the midriff can all be treated. Mesotherapy dissolves cellulite and unwanted inches but doesn't require patients to take days or weeks off work. It is easier on the patient and more precise than liposuction, and because it is more precise, it can target problems such as cellulite that liposuction cannot affect. Liposuction removes fat cells through a suctioning procedure. Mesotherapy, on the other hand, employs medications that break down the fat-cell membrane and let the fat out. These medications are injected into the mesoderm—the middle (fat) layer of the skin. Once broken down, the displaced fat enters the bloodstream. There it is either burned as energy or excreted. To hasten this, doctors recommend injections of multivitamins and high-fiber diets.

Now a new and important form of this therapy called lipodissolve has been developed. Lipodissolve uses injections of phosphotiylcholine/deoxycholate (pc/dc). Many practitioners have further developed the pc/dc lipodissolve treatment and some combine it with ultrasound and/or endermologie to get the best results.

Lipodissolve injections cause little discomfort because exceptionally tiny needles are used. However the medication burns likes fire ants under the skin in the treated area for about an hour, though this is greatly diminished by wearing tight clothing such as a girdle or bicycle pants. Bruising and swelling persists for a few days and the discomfort can last for a few weeks. For most people, the little

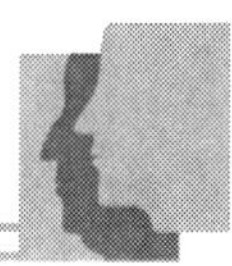

bit of pain is worth it because results start to be visible in as little as 72 hours and are cumulative with successive treatments. I find four treatments work for most people. Mesotherapy was originally developed in France in the 1950s by Dr. Michel Pistor and in 1988 it was accepted as part of the standard armentarium of French medicine. It was introduced to North America in 1998 by Dr. Lionel Bissoon, who learned the technique in France. His most famous patient is singer Roberta Flack (famous for "Killing Me Softly With His Song") who felt that her extra pounds were indeed killing her softly. With mesotherapy, exercise and a reformed diet, Flack lost 40 pounds

Closer to home, take the example of my patient, Jane, who is now 49. She had three liposuction procedures and got great results—for liposuction. But some irregularities remained and they were impossible to remove further with liposuction. With just two sessions of mesotherapy (combined in alternate two-week sessions with endermologie, a suction assisted massage), the irregularities *melted* away, leaving her thrilled. "I'm so glad science brings on these new therapies," she told me, "just when aging forces me to need them."

Denise is a 39-year-old secretary. Originally a size 13, she's now a size 9, thanks to mesotherapy and endermologie.

Indra, at the age of 60, looks great and participates in ballroom dancing. Her upper abdomen would not respond to exercise and dieting, but with two treatments of mesotherapy, her abdomen is significantly slimmed.

Overall I'm delighted this technique works so well. I'm a 21-year veteran of liposuction procedures, and I find there is a role for both mesotherapy and liposuction. I'd been accustomed to doing up to eight very physical liposuction procedures a week and they've taken their toll—the constant, repetitive movement leaving me with a chronic shoulder injury. Lipodissolve and laser lipolysis have allowed me to leave that problem behind.

The American TV program *20/20* looked at mesotherapy in 2003. The program followed two persons, patients of the featured practitioner Dr. Lionel Bissoon. According to Bissoon's records, Josselyne Herman-Saccio, a 35-year-old mother of two, was able to lose three or four inches from her waist and three or four in her hips in six weeks. Katie Noonan-Ewald, a 32-year-old business executive, lost 24 inches from her waist and another 12 inches from her hips, legs, and saddlebag area in 12 weeks.

Although injections may seem strange to some patients, plastic surgeons have been using injections for years. Some scars—keloids and hypertrophic scars for example—literally melt away with injections of cortisone. Mesotherapy injections are not that different.

Controversy nonetheless surrounds some of the agents employed in the mesotherapy technique. An investigation by the television show *60 minutes* found phosphotidylcholine, one of the ingredients that break down the fat cell membrane, has been banned in Brazil. But this restriction understandably arose when people began using the medicine in an unsafe manner. For example, the procedures were so popular in Brazil, they were being done in the back rooms of hair salons. Any medication, when not used safely, can be dangerous. The company making this medication voluntarily withdrew it from the Brazil market.

Mesotherapy is not simply for those with too much money and not enough motivation. Nor is it just for the vain. Many of my clients are devoted athletes who exercise hours everyday. Unfortunately, fat happens, and it happens to hockey players and ballerinas, too. The body is built so that you cannot directly burn the fat on top of a muscle by exercising the muscle below it.

Mesotherapy currently costs about $500 to $1,000 per injection area. However, some physicians offer packages that make treatments more economical. For example, a package of four treatments, four endermologie treatments and a body suit, which might normally cost $200, may be packaged at $2350.

Meanwhile, many doctors are experimenting with other mesotherapy "recipes" and we can expect even faster and more favorable

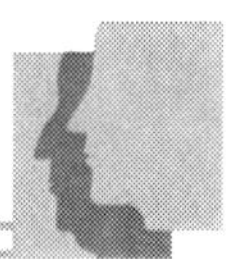

results in the future. Expect to see more studies published shortly.

## Breast Implants

Breast implants (also known as *breast enlargement* or *augmentation*) are saline- or silicone-filled bags slid in between the breast tissue and the chest muscles, or between the chest muscles and the chest wall. Patients are normally able to get out of bed a day or two after the surgery is done, but are not usually able to bathe for three to seven days. A few days to a week after the operation, they may feel well enough to return to work, but shouldn't do any vigorous exercise for two to three weeks. The cost is around $3,000 but again, it varies by surgeon and location.

In the last decade, breast implants took a bad rap because of reported side effects. Scientifically, the only side effects that have been demonstrated have been some leakage of silicone out of silicone implants. These side effects are rare but can occur. Improved breast implants have since been developed and this rare problem has become even rarer.

## Breast Reduction

Breast reduction is done by removing excess breast tissue and skin and reshaping the breast. Women may seek breast reduction not only to alter their appearance but also to reduce back pain and reduce the limitations placed on their activities caused by large breasts.

## The Tummy Tuck

Also known as abdominoplasty, a tummy tuck removes excess skin from the abdominal area and tightens the abdominal muscles. The procedure results in a flatter, smoother stomach. As with liposuction, the purpose of a tummy tuck is to reshape an area of the body rather than to reduce body weight.

Again, this procedure is not used to treat obesity. Its intention is wholly cosmetic. In truth, surgery is rarely used to treat obesity and most doctors will consider it only for people who have not been able to lose weight with other treatments and who are at high risk for developing other health problems because of their weight.

## Treatment for Unwanted Veins

Varicose veins are twisted, enlarged veins near the surface of the skin. They most commonly develop in the legs and ankles. Smaller varicose veins may be referred to as spider veins. Varicose veins are visible through the skin and appear dark blue, swollen, and twisted.

Varicose veins are thought to be related to defective valves in the circulatory system or to weakened and stretched vein walls, although it is not clear whether valve problems are a cause or an effect of the weakened, stretched vein walls. However, the result is an inability of the veins to keep blood flowing against gravity, up toward the heart. Blood pools in the legs and pressure builds up in the veins.

People may be more likely to develop varicose veins because of their genetics, the aging process, or hormone changes. Varicose veins may also result from conditions such as obesity, pregnancy or having an occupation that requires you to stand for long periods of time. These increase the pressure on the leg veins.

Varicose veins are common and are not usually a sign of a serious medical problem. However, in some cases, varicose veins can signal a problem in the deeper veins. Deep vein problems require evaluation and possibly treatment. For more information, see the topic Deep Leg-Vein Thrombosis.

### *Symptoms*

You may not have symptoms with varicose veins. Most people identify varicose veins by the appearance of twisted, swollen, bluish veins just beneath the skin. If you have symptoms of varicose veins, they tend to be mild and may include:

- A dull ache, burning, or heaviness in the legs. These symptoms

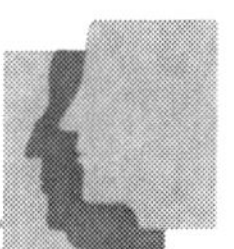

may be more noticeable late in the day or after you have been sitting or standing for a long time.

♦ Mild swelling, usually involving the feet and ankles only.

♦ Itching skin over the varicose vein.

More severe symptoms or complications may include:

♦ A build-up of fluid (edema) and swelling in the leg.

♦ Significant swelling and calf pain after sitting or standing for a long time.

♦ Skin color changes (stasis pigmentation) around the ankles and lower legs.

♦ Dry, stretched, swollen, itching, or scaling skin.

♦ Superficial thrombophlebitis, (inflammation of the superficial veins of the legs)

♦ Open sores (ulcerations).

♦ Bleeding after a minor trauma.

Symptoms of varicose veins may become more severe a few days before and during a woman's menstrual period, suggesting a hormonal relationship.

### *Treatment*

Depending on the specifics of the case, the goals of varicose vein treatment may be improved appearance, reduced symptoms or the prevention of complications.

Doctors recommend home treatment (especially exercising, wearing compression stockings, and elevating the legs) as a first step for varicose veins. This may be all you need to relieve the symptoms. If you are not satisfied with the results of home treatment and are thinking about having surgery or sclerotherapy (a technique that involves injecting a chemical into the unwanted veins), you will want to know which treatment is best for you. No single approach is best for treating all varicose veins. Surgery tends to work better for larger veins, while sclerotherapy may be the best approach for smaller varicose veins and spider veins.

Many treatment methods (such as all types of surgery, sclerotherapy, laser, and radiofrequency ablation) may scar or discolor the skin. Deep vein problems or problems with the "perforating" veins that connect the deep and superficial veins, can result in varicose veins that are difficult to treat. Sclerotherapy or conventional varicose vein surgery often cannot help because these treatments do not correct the underlying problem.

Sclerotherapy or ligation (tying off of veins), may be considered if symptoms and complications (such as pain, inflammation of the skin, and ulcers) develop or continue to get worse despite home treatment. In these cases, treatment may be necessary to remove the damaged veins, ameliorate complications or correct an underlying problem that is causing the varicose veins. The size of your varicose veins will affect your treatment options. Generally, larger varicose veins are treated with surgery (ligation and stripping). Smaller varicose veins and spider veins are usually treated with sclerotherapy or laser therapy. As newer techniques in sclerotherapy are developed and become more widely available, their use to treat larger varicose veins may increase. Laser and radiofrequency ablation is another technique that has recently been approved by the U.S. Food and Drug Administration (FDA) and is sometimes used to treat large varicose veins.

Some people may want to improve how their legs look, even though their varicose veins are not causing other problems. In these cases, surgery or sclerotherapy may be appropriate where the person does not have other health problems that make these treatments risky.

## Treatments for Cellulite

Cellulite is that bumpy, orange-peel-like fat bemoaned by women everywhere. Sometimes referred to as "cottage cheese thighs," what might look like an alien life-form burrowing beneath your skin is simply normal fat. It looks bumpy because it's pushing through the connective tissues that usually keep it distributed evenly beneath your skin. The total amount of fat in your body, your age, and your

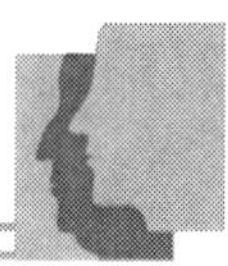

genetic predisposition (blame your parents!) all combine to determine if you'll be saddled with cellulite or not.

While it's impossible to know just how many women are driven batty by cellulite, scientists say that about 85% of women have some. It is a surprisingly equal-opportunity annoyance, appearing on thin and heavy women alike. Everyone wants an instant fix, a magic pill. There just isn't one.

Diet and exercise, however, remain your best bet. Be patient: it can take at least six months of hard work to see any improvement. Be sure to add so-called resistance training—weight lifting is an example—to your routine. The stronger muscles it will help build underneath your fat deposits can help smooth out the area overall. Still, even with good diet and exercise, some cellulite may remain. At some point you have to accept that you have done all you can.

Recently, mesotherapy and endermologie have been used to significantly alter this problem. Some lasers and deep heating machines have also been used, with variable results. Think of them as turbo-powered cellulite removal.

Though plenty of women are looking for a quick cellulite fix in a jar, lotions and potions have yielded little satisfaction. Over the last few years, a handful of cellulite creams have stormed the market, with pseudo-scientific infomercials flooding TV screens nationwide touting a dramatic reduction in the appearance of cellulite by increasing blood flow to the affected areas. Do they work? Unfortunately, no. Cellulite creams appear to be more hype than fact. People need to remember that the beauty industry can make claims based on anecdotal evidence that have no scientific or medical backing whatsoever. A double-blind study published in the September 1999 issue of the British *Journal of Plastic and Reconstructive Surgery* put the creams to the test. After 12 weeks, only three of the 17 women in the study reported even the slightest improvement.

Many drugstores stock a pre-packaged, over-the-counter pill called Cellasene. Cellasene, which contains a mixture of herbs such as ginkgo biloba, sweet clover, and grape-seed oil, as well as non-herbal ingredients, claims to improve capillary circulation, inhibit collagen breakdown (which helps keeps skin firm and elastic), and support healthy connective tissue, thereby reducing the appearance of cellulite. But when British researchers evaluated Cellasene in a November 1999 study, their results were lukewarm. In this study, one group of women took Cellasene and one group took a placebo pill for two months. There was no noticeable improvement in the cellulite in either group. In addition, some doctors caution that the high level of iodine in the pills may lead to thyroid problems.

Even massaging cellulite away through a procedure called endermologie often shows no noticeable difference in before-and-after photographs. During endermologie or Dermosonic™, available only at physicians' offices, a vacuum-like device deeply massages the areas where there is noticeable cellulite. The technique purports to redistribute the fat under the connective tissues and to lead to a smoother, more balanced appearance. It has a qualified endorsement from the Food and Drug Administration. The same British study that evaluated cellulite creams also tested the effects of an endermologie program that included twice-weekly treatments for 12 weeks. About one third of those treated felt their cellulite had improved. Dermosonic™ is similar to endermologie but adds ultrasound to fat reduction treatments.

Some doctors do report a better result when they combine endermologie with mesotherapy and I am generally in agreement. And while we physicians continue to investigate the best techniques available, scientists continue their search for the genetic key that might explain why some people get cellulite and others do not.

## Tattoos

Tattoos can usually be completely or almost completely erased with four to 30 sessions of laser treatment over several weeks or months. Usually some skin color changes occur in the treated area. Rarely,

laser treatment may make the ink in the tattoo darker and harder to remove. The long-term results may not be evident for several months.

Generally, tattoo removal requires a high energy Nd/YAG, alexandrite or ruby laser. One of the most rewarding parts of cosmetic practice is to erase tattoos for former gang members and prostitutes. Such procedures effectively free people who would otherwise be tied by these disfigurements to the lives they used to live.

# Chapter 5

# Your Hair

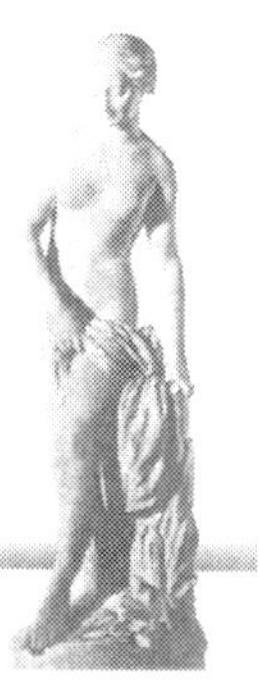

## MEET YOUR HAIR

We all have hair, which seems to be left over from an earlier stage of evolution, when it served to protect us just as it does other mammals. You might be surprised to learn that you have just as many hairs on your body as a gorilla. The difference is that your hair is much finer than that of a gorilla, something you're probably happy about. An abundance of body hair might be an impediment for creatures like us who have found other ways to protect ourselves. Most of our remaining hair is on our heads, where it stands between our brains and the sun.

Hair is a protein that grows out of the hair follicles in your skin. A hair follicle produces a hair for a period of time—typically many months—before the hair stops growing, falls out and a new hair grows.

## HAIR CARE

Most of the threat to healthy hair occurs outside in the parching sun or harsh cold. Regardless of the weather, the sun's UV rays still pound down on your hair. Heat, severe cold, UV rays, and chlorinated water can be a nightmare combination for your hair if you don't take the right precautions.

For starters, look around for a conditioner containing products that protect against UV rays. Hair is as sensitive as skin when it comes to UV rays, and it needs to be covered. If you can't find a conditioner with sunscreen in it, just brush a dab of SPF-fortified lotion into your hair, use a spray on, or wear a hat.

If you can't resist a little sun effect on your locks, at least refrain from outside help. Hair lightening products generally contain peroxide or metallic salt, both of which are bad news for your hair. These products can backfire, turning what you hoped would be natural highlights into pink or orange streaks. Combining metallic salt residue with perm chemicals, even trace amounts, can destroy your scalp, turning your "do" into clumps in the shower drain. If you have to have some help sunning your hair, try a little bit of lemon juice, but don't use anything harsher than that.

And of course, there's the matter of chlorine. As unbelievable as the horror stories seem, they can be all too real. To avoid serious issues, don't get near a pool too soon before or after a perm. The green-hair story is not a myth. Perm chemicals can react to chlorine in funky ways, leaving hair green, bleached, fried, or otherwise ruined. Even if your hair isn't permed, chlorine can be damaging. Condition your hair before getting in the pool, and wash and condition as soon as you get out. If you plan to spend a lot of time in the water, find a hair clarifier, a stronger-than-normal shampoo designed to remove toxins. Clarifiers are too harsh to use everyday, but using them twice a week should counteract the brittle, dried-out effect chlorine can have.

Just remember that when you change your hair's routine or expose your hair to more than it's used to, you have to compensate with that much more prevention and care. Keep your hair clean, conditioned, and free of outside agents that can react to too much sun and too much water.

## Folliculitis

Each strand of body hair grows from within a very small sac or cavity called a follicle, which lies beneath the skin. Infection of the hair follicles is called folliculitis and is usually caused by bacteria or fungi. Certain chemicals—and, rarely, medications or viruses—can also cause folliculitis. Many people first notice folliculitis on areas where clothing rubs against the body, such as the arms, legs, thighs, and buttocks.

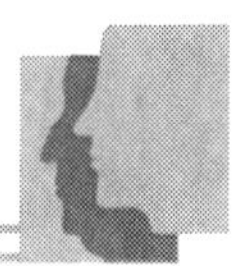

Folliculitis can also occur on the scalp and face. The hair follicles of men's beards are especially prone to this infection.

Normally, the skin has various types of bacteria and fungi on its surface. Folliculitis usually develops when some event causes the bacteria or fungi to grow into the skin. This can occur:

- ♦ After sitting in water that contains bacteria or fungi.
- ♦ As a result of poor personal hygiene, especially related to irregular bathing or crowded living conditions.
- ♦ From wearing tight-fitting clothes (jeans, athletic clothes, or underwear) that can trap bacteria. If you sweat while wearing tight clothing, your pores open and the trapped bacteria can more easily enter the skin and grow.
- ♦ When taking antibiotics or steroid creams for long periods. These medications often destroy protective bacteria, leaving the skin unable to fight the bacteria or fungi that cause folliculitis.
- ♦ From clogged pores, often caused by cosmetics or dry skin.
- ♦ From open wounds, such as cuts, scrapes, or surgical incisions. If an infection develops in a wound, it can spread to nearby hair follicles. This can occur after shaving.
- ♦ From having a long-term disease such as diabetes or HIV (the virus that causes AIDS) that prevents your body from fighting infection normally.

Folliculitis caused by bacteria or fungi can spread when you don't wash your hands after touching an infected area. The infection may spread from one part of your body to another or to other people. Folliculitis can also spread from infected personal items such as towels or clothes. The severity of folliculitis varies. Mild (superficial) folliculitis infections are close to the skin surface and usually heal on their own in about two weeks. Severe (deep) folliculitis infections last longer, are deep in the skin, cause pain and may leave scars.

Folliculitis caused by fungi usually lasts longer—six weeks or more—than folliculitis caused by bacteria. Some types of fungal folliculitis can cause scarring and become a persistent problem that needs long-term treatment. Sometimes folliculitis occurs along with or progresses to acne or other deep skin infections such as a boil (furuncle). A carbuncle is larger and more painful than a boil and can also result from folliculitis. If you have a carbuncle, you may also have a fever and feel ill. Some other skin conditions have symptoms similar to folliculitis.

Early treatment of folliculitis with antibiotic ointments or antifungal creams usually clears up the condition. Special shampoos are also available to treat folliculitis that occurs on the scalp or beard. When mild folliculitis is caused by bacteria, it may often be treated with antibiotic ointments or creams such as bacitracin, polymyxin B sulfate (Polysporin), clindomycin, erythromycin, or mupirocin (Bactroban). Topical antiseptic cleansers such as povidone-iodine or chlorhexidine may also be used. Mild cases of folliculitis sometimes heal on their own. However, folliculitis may return or get worse. If you have symptoms of folliculitis that spread or return, see a health professional for proper treatment.

Oral antibiotics are usually successful in clearing up deeper, more severe folliculitis infections. A fluid sample from an infected follicle may be analyzed to help your doctor determine the specific cause of your folliculitis in order to determine which medication is best for you.

Deeper or more severe bacterial infections are usually treated with oral antibiotics in the form of pills. Cloxacillin, erythromycin, and cephalexin (such as Keflex) are used to treat many infections. Ciprofloxacin (such as Cipro) and ofloxacin (such as Floxin) are used when specific types of bacteria are causing infection.

Folliculitis caused by a fungus is most often treated with antifungal pills such as fluconazole (Diflucan), griseofulvin (for example, Fluvican U/F or Gris-PEG), itraconazole (Sporanox), or terbinafine (Lamasil). Sometimes, anti-inflammatory pills (corticosteroids) or medications may also be used.

If folliculitis occurs on the scalp or beard area, you may be advised

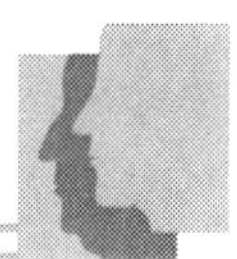

to use special shampoos that contain selenium sulfide 2.5%, selenium 1%, or 50% propylene glycol (such as Selsun Blue).

Self-care is also an important part of treatment for folliculitis. Preventing the development and spread of folliculitis is important, as is treating the symptoms.

Home treatment for folliculitis includes:

♦ Using a soap that kills bacteria (an antibacterial soap) to wash the infected area. If the infection is on the scalp or beard area, use a special shampoo containing selenium or propylene glycol (such as Selsun Blue). Your doctor may also prescribe a ketoconazde topical (Nizoral Topical) medicated shampoo to use regularly.

♦ Applying warm wet compresses three to six times a day to help folliculitis heal faster and stop the itching or pain. To make a compress, moisten a clean cloth or piece of gauze with warm water. Place it over the infected area until it begins to cool (usually five to 10 minutes). Burow's solution or white vinegar solution may be used instead of water. Wash your hands before applying a compress.

There are a number of things you can do to prevent folliculitis from developing, spreading or recurring.

♦ Bathe or shower regularly. Changing clothes and bathing are particularly helpful shortly after exercise or work that involves chemicals. This will help avoid trapping bacteria or chemicals that can enter the pores of your skin. A mild antibacterial soap may also be helpful.

♦ Avoid sharing towels, washcloths, or other personal items; use a clean washcloth and towel each time you bathe if you have folliculitis.

♦ Don't scratch infected areas. Organisms that cause folliculitis can be carried under your fingernails and spread to other areas of your body or to other people.

♦ Wash your hands often, especially when you or someone you are caring for has a skin infection. Pay special attention to cleaning under your fingernails.

If you have folliculitis, avoid shaving the infected area. If you must shave, change the razor blade each time or use ointments and lotions that remove hair without shaving (depilatory creams and lotions). These products are not suggested for men as a substitute for shaving their beards because the products can irritate the skin if used more often than every 36 hours.

Wear loose-fitting clothing. Tighter clothes trap sweat and bacteria on your body. Avoid using oils on your skin. Oils can cause bacteria to be trapped in the pores of your skin and can cause folliculitis to develop or recur.

Use a mild deodorant.

Avoid public hot tubs or spas. When you do use them, shower immediately and wash with antibacterial soap. If you own your own hot tub, keep it clean. Follow the instructions provided by the hot tub's manufacturer.

If you have folliculitis, call a health professional if it spreads or keeps coming back. If you develop other symptoms, such as fever over 101°F (38.33°C), redness, swelling, warmth, or increased pain over the infected area, you should seek medical advice immediately.

## Unwanted Hair

Hair does not appear on our bodies for cosmetic purposes. It occurs as vestiges of earlier stages of evolution or grows naturally as a protection against cold, skin injury, etc. For example, if a man has a cut on his face away from his normal shaving area, he may find whiskers growing near the cut where no hairs grew before. This may be attributed to the body's attempt to protect the damaged area with hair. In response to fashion, we may wish to shed some of our hair. Unfortunately, trying too hard can cause health problems.

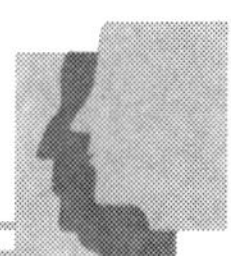

## Razor Bumps

For the faces of men and legs of women, razor bumps are a common and treatable nuisance. Normally, hair grows to the surface of the skin in a tube called a follicle, without touching the skin itself. If your beard is naturally thick and curly, or if your follicles grow out at oblique angles to the skin's surface, shaving can give the hairs sharp ends. If the sharp ends penetrate the skin, the body reacts as if to any foreign object, such as a splinter. This can lead to a very red, pimple-like bump. Here are some changes in your shaving routine that can help reduce this problem:

♦ Take a warm shower for at least two minutes before shaving to soften your beard. Hairs will cut more easily and the severed ends will be duller, making penetration of the skin less likely.

♦ Use a razor that does not shave as closely or try an electric razor that is not set at the closest setting. Apply a lubricated shaving gel made for use with electric razors.

♦ Choose a razor with a single blade. Double- or triple-bladed razors cut hair shafts so far down that they may recoil much farther back into the follicles. The hairs then may penetrate the follicle and cause a reaction in the surrounding skin.

♦ To dislodge hairs that may be starting to grow into the skin, use a short-bristled toothbrush. Using a circular motion, gently brush the parts of your face that are prone to razor bumps once or twice daily.

♦ Avoid aftershaves or colognes, which may irritate your skin. Instead, try a moisturizer containing lactic acid or glycolic acid to help soften the hairs.

Be patient. It may take several days or even a few weeks to see improvement.

If these suggestions do not work, you may as a last resort want to consider alternatives to shaving, such as depilatories and electrolysis. Occasionally red bumps are a sign of an infection. If the bumps do not resolve or improve, see your doctor or a dermatologist or try a prescription chemical treatment.

One of the most powerful and popular treatments for razor bumps is Eflornithine, a topical medication for external use only. Available in the United States, it has yet to be approved in Canada. The secret to its success is continuous application, even if there are no immediate results. Reduction in facial hair occurs gradually. Improvement may be seen as early as four to eight weeks of treatment, though it may take longer in some individuals. If no improvement is seen after six months of use, treatment with Eflornithine topical should be discontinued. Hair growth may return to pretreatment levels approximately eight weeks after discontinuation of treatment with Eflornithine topical.

Eflornithine interferes with a natural chemical in the hair follicles of the skin. This results in slower hair growth where Eflornithine topical is applied. The manufacturer advertises Enflornithine topical as useful for the reduction of unwanted facial hair in women, but it is used for both men and women. It does not permanently remove hair or "cure" unwanted facial hair.

## Electrolysis

Electrolysis is the removal of unwanted hair through the means of a needle inserted into the follicle. There are three different methods (modalities) used to accomplish this:

♦ Short Wave: A high frequency radio energy, which sets up a rapid oscillation or vibration in the cells of the follicle producing heat. Using this method, the hair tissue is then cauterized.

♦ Galvanic: The galvanic method uses direct current to produce sodium hydroxide in the follicle, which then acts chemically to annihilate the hair tissue.

♦ Blend: The blend method combines both the *short wave* and *galvanic* modalities. The oscillation of the high frequency radio energy produces heated sodium hydroxide that destroys the hair tissue.

One of the greatest fears of someone considering this process is

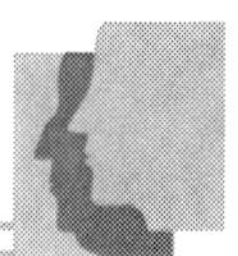

that there is pain involved. But although there may be some discomfort, this varies with the individual undergoing the treatment. Electrolysis is a safe, permanent process of hair removal that can be applied to anyone. Men and women can both benefit. If you feel that unwanted hair is in any way a nuisance or an embarrassment, then electrolysis is definitely for you.

When choosing a practitioner, there are important questions to ask:

- How much training have they had?
- Are their certificates visible?
- How long have they been in business?
- What type of needles do they use?
- Will they work on both men and women?
- Do they take a full history before treating you?
- Do they provide after-treatment care and suggestions?
- Can you call them later with questions?
- Do you feel comfortable in their office and with them?
- How do they bill for their work? Is it in office time or working time?

Although there are many reasons to choose electrolysis over other methods of hair removal such as tweezing, shaving or waxing, there is one reason that stands above all the others: it's permanent. By using the electrolysis method, you will see that unwanted hair will be removed safely, and permanently.

### Chemical Removal of Hair

Chemicals to remove hair are nothing new. Products like Nair and other depilatories have been on the market for years. But they can be harsh on the skin—sometimes burning the area treated. You might want to try other home remedies or turn to a prescription chemical treatment.

## Laser Hair Removal

Laser hair-removal (the use of a powerful light-emitting technology to treat hair) is unseating electrolysis as the preferred method of permanent hair removal—especially as the technology improves. Though this procedure is a popular choice with women who have difficulty removing their unwanted hair on their legs, contrary to popular belief, a few zaps of a laser doesn't mean you can totally retire your razor. What the laser can do, however, is to reduce the amount of hair you have and perhaps lead to some permanent hair removal. In addition, it can lighten the color of the hair and decrease its thickness.

Laser hair removal takes about an hour for both legs. As the laser is moved over your legs, the light passes through your skin and gets absorbed by the melanin (pigment) in the hair follicles. Although no one knows exactly how lasers reduce hair growth, the most popular theory is that the heat generated by the laser affects the hair growth centre in the follicle. Over the next two months, hairs gradually fall out. For most people, the pain—similar to a rubber band snapping on the skin—is quite tolerable. If you're very sensitive, however, your doctor can apply a topical anesthetic cream to numb the area.

Before you sign up for laser hair removal, though, take into account your natural hair and skin color, as the treatment tends to work best on fair-skinned people with dark hair. If you're tanned or have a darker skin tone, the laser gets absorbed by the pigment in the skin and doesn't reach the hair follicle, limiting the effect of the treatment and potentially damaging the skin. The procedure doesn't seem to work very well on light-haired people either, whose hair contains little melanin.

You should keep in mind that at least six treatments, three to six weeks apart, may be needed to achieve a meaningful reduction in the amount of hair on your legs (or elsewhere). Most studies have shown a 90% hair reduction by that time. After that, you'll need to wait a year to see the full effect of the treatment. Hair growth-cycles are about six months long, so it's best to wait through two growth-cycles

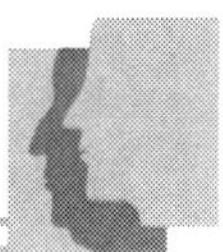

to assess the final results.

Since the area treated will be sensitive for a few days, it is wise to wear both protective clothing and sun block whenever you're outside. In addition, plan to limit your sun exposure for a day or two after the treatment, as you can expect some slight swelling and redness. These side effects should disappear within a day and can be soothed with ice or a mild anti-inflammatory cream. Rarer side effects include peeling, blistering, and burning of the skin as well as brown spots and slight loss of pigment in areas where the laser has been used.

Taking all of these factors into account, if you have your heart set on total and permanent hair removal, electrolysis—where an electrical pulse is used to permanently stop the hair follicles from producing hair—may be a better bet than going under the laser. Nonetheless laser hair removal has, in my opinion, supplanted electrolysis in many situations because it is easier, less painful, and less tedious.

## HAIR ANALYSIS

If you do experience health conditions that might impact your hair, your doctor might prescribe a hair analysis. Samples of hair can be analyzed under a microscope and by using various chemical tests. Hair analysis can help diagnose some health problems (such as a fungal infection ) or can be used to detect illegal drug use (such as the use of PCP ). In addition, a hair sample can be used to analyze DNA, which can help determine whether two people are likely to be blood relatives. This often finds application in paternity cases. Forensic hair analysis can help identify a criminal or exonerate an innocent person by evaluating hair structure and DNA.

Common uses of hair analysis include:

♦ Diagnosing fungal diseases that affect the skin, including athlete's foot, ringworm of the scalp, and ringworm of the groin (jock itch).

♦ Helping to provide DNA evidence for criminal and paternity cases. For DNA testing, the root of one hair is needed to analyze DNA and to establish a person's genetic makeup.

Less common and/or controversial uses of hair analysis include:

♦ Testing for illegal drug use, such as the use of cocaine, marijuana, or PCP.

♦ Testing for the presence of heavy metals in the body, such as lead, mercury, and arsenic.

♦ Screening for nutritional deficiencies in the body. Hair analysis cannot reliably determine the need for vitamin and mineral supplements.

♦ Screening for undiagnosed diseases, such as cancer or kidney failure.

A hair typically grows for many months before it falls out. During that time, changes in your body—including diet, health and the ingestion of chemicals—may be reflected in the composition of your hair. But it takes weeks for a hair sample to reflect what has occurred in the body. Because hair grows slowly, hair samples do not show recent changes in the body such as drug use within the previous few days.

If you have a hair analysis done, the laboratory will give you specific instructions on how to prepare your hair. Hair preparation and the part of your body from which the hair is taken varies. Generally, your hair should be washed and free of any hair care products.

If hair samples are being obtained to detect illegal drug use, you should be prepared to list all medications (both prescription and nonprescription), herbal supplements, vitamins, and any other substances you are taking, because they may interfere with testing. You may need to sign a form (consent form) that says you understand the risks of the test and agree to have it done. As you read the consent form, ask your doctor any questions you have about the test and discuss any worries you may have about your need for the test, the risks of the test, or how it will be done.

Hair analysis is done by collecting a hair sample and sending it to

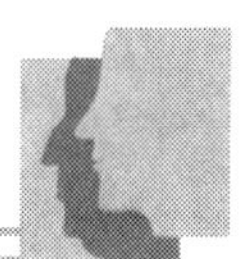

a laboratory: Hair samples are taken from a specific part of the body, such as from the back of the scalp by the neck or from the pubic area. Hair samples are generally collected from the section of the hair closest to the skin. Hair close to the skin or scalp includes the most recent growth, which provides the most accurate information about what has occurred recently in the body. Hair samples are washed in special chemicals before testing.

Samples of hair used for drug testing will probably be obtained by laboratory personnel. Getting a good sample from the right part of the body is essential to obtain accurate results. Hair samples for DNA analysis will be gathered by laboratory personnel or law enforcement officials. For DNA testing, the hair must include the root. This requires that the hair be plucked, not cut.

If you are collecting your own hair sample, follow the instructions given to you by the laboratory. Generally you will be asked to:

- Clip a small sample of your hair (usually about a spoonful) from the nape of your neck. The sample should be onein. (2.5 cm) to 1.5 in. (3.8 cm) long and should include the new growth closest to the scalp.
- Put the clippings in a plastic bag and seal it.
- Send the samples to the laboratory along with information about the type of hair treatments you have used, including shampoos, conditioners, colorings, bleaches, and permanents. Information about your age, height, weight, sex, and whether you smoke may also be requested by the laboratory.

If you are collecting your own sample:

- Clean the infected area of the skin with rubbing alcohol (70% alcohol) to remove bacteria.
- Clip hair samples from the infected area on the scalp or beard.
- Pluck out any remaining hair stubs with tweezers. Fungus is usually found at the base of a hair shaft.
- Place the sample in a sterile container that you get from the laboratory or your health professional.

There is generally no pain or discomfort associated with this test. However, if you have to pluck a hair for a DNA test, this may c ause some minor discomfort. Hair analysis itself has no risks or complications.

The results of hair analysis are usually complete within three weeks. You or your doctor will receive a report listing the levels of minerals and heavy metals in your hair. Several factors need to be considered before testing for heavy metal exposure or your nutritional state.

There is no standard procedure for cutting, washing, and analyzing hair. Different labs may report different results from the same hair sample. In fact, the same lab may report different results for separate hairs from a common sample. It is difficult to interpret a hair analysis for the presence of heavy metals or nutritional deficiencies.

The significance of most of the findings from hair analysis is unclear. What the hair sample contains is determined not only by nutrition and internal metabolism but also by external substances. Air pollution, mineral content of the water supply, exposure to industrial waste, shampoos, hair dyes, hair sprays, permanents, and bleaches may raise or lower the levels of certain minerals in the hair. In addition, the use of medications such as birth control pills can change the mineral concentration of hair. For most trace minerals, what really constitutes normal or significant deviations from normal is not known.

Most professionals believe that hair analysis to detect heavy metals and nutrients is unreliable. Standards for testing do not exist. Any hair analysis to detect the presence or absence of minerals, nutrients, or toxic metals in the body should be confirmed by testing blood and urine samples.

Factors that can affect the results of hair analysis include:

The area of the body from which the hair sample was taken.

- Your age
- Your hair color

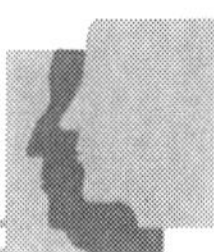

- Your race
- The rate of hair growth
- The use of hair products, such as hair colors and sprays
- External environmental factors, such as where you live and work.

Some natural health and homeopathic companies offer hair analysis by mail order. The reports are mailed to you along with recommendations for taking various vitamin and mineral supplements. Sometimes these same companies sell vitamin and mineral supplements. The test results may be accurate. However, you need to evaluate the results of the tests the same as you would for any health procedure. If you have any questions, talk with your health professional.

Although hair analysis is being done more frequently to test for illegal drug use (such as the use of cocaine, marijuana, or PCP), it is not widely available. Drug screening is more commonly done on blood or urine samples.

# Chapter 6

# Some Final Thoughts

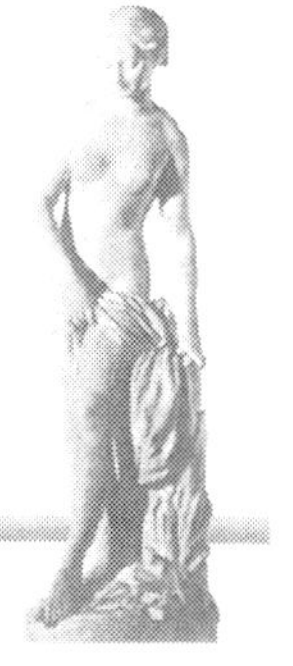

## Cosmetic Surgery: The Trends

Cosmetic surgery used to be considered something of a "last resort." If you were in your 60s and just couldn't bear the image of your aging body in the mirror, you'd contact a plastic surgeon and hope that his scalpel could miraculously take a decade or more off your appearance. But as the popularity of cosmetic surgery spreads across the country, more people are walking into doctors' offices knowing exactly the look they want, often specifically requesting a certain actress' nose or lips. These days, people of all ages seem to be rushing to go under the knife. According to the American Society for Aesthetic Plastic Surgery, over 10.2 million cosmetic surgical and nonsurgical procedures were performed in the United States in 2008. Canadian figures are about 10% of that. And the trend is clearly moving toward increasingly younger patients and less invasive procedures.

It's common to see people in their 30s having their eyelids surgically done, because that's really the first thing to age. In their 40s, they might start thinking about facelifts. Add to that the present fashion for midriff-revealing tops and low-riding jeans—no wonder the demand for tummy tucks and abdominal liposuction is surging as well.

Among baby boomers in particular, plastic surgery appears to be out of the closet, with the 35- to 50-year-old group accounting for 44% of the cosmetic procedures performed in 2001. And cosmetic surgery is no longer the exclusive domain of women. The number of procedures performed on men rose to more than one million in 2001, or about 12% of the total, often because men believe that a more youthful appearance offers a career advantage.

No region of the world exemplifies this search for perfection more than the Los Angeles area. There's no question that Southern California—with the lifestyle and attitudes that prevail there—is the cosmetic surgery capital of the world. The people of L.A. place great importance on their physical appearance. Within the 5.6 square miles of Beverly Hills are more plastic surgeons and out-patient surgery centers, not to mention more dermatologists and hair salons, than in any comparable area in the world.

It was in L.A. that doctors first gave prospective patients a computer-enhanced image of how they'll look *after* surgery. People can e-mail photos of themselves to a surgeons office, where they are fine-tuned by a software program that can remove bags, sculpt the chin line, remove the bump from the nose, and erase wrinkles. In minutes, the "new look" can be emailed back to the individuals for viewing on their own computer screen. Not that this service is limited to Hollywood. I can do it in my own office in Edmonton, Alberta.

If you're in the market for age regression after reading all of this, there's plenty to choose from, including new and evolving procedures. For example, while patients with bags under their eyes have benefited for years from the removal of fat in that area, surgeons have recently begun redistributing the existing fat in patients who have a groove or depression under the heavy bags, using that fat to eliminate bulges and puffiness, and producing a more smoothly contoured lower lid.

Doctors also do "cleavoplasties" on women who have undergone breast augmentation and feel that the area between their breasts appears bony and unattractive. In these women, body fat taken from the thighs or abdomen is placed in the area over the sternum to improve the contour between the breasts. And I mustn't overlook "mommy makeovers," which have become quite common. Meanwhile, if thongs are your thing, you can have your buttocks augmented for a rounder, fuller look, which could involve the use of buttock implants,

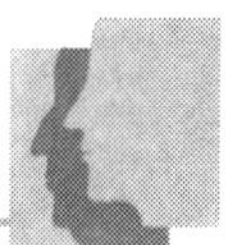

or "micro-fat grafting" in which fat is removed from one part of the body and injected into the buttocks.

For those who opt for any type of cosmetic procedure, the surgeon's tools have improved, too. They have access to better pain medications and better drugs to help people relax and sleep. The anesthetics are safer and shorter-acting, too. And so many procedures are now "outpatient": you can have your nose done at 7 A.M. and be home for dinner.

Barring an unfortunate condition that might force you to have a procedure done, the final decision of whether or not to pursue cosmetic surgery or a related treatment is up to you. I've written this book so you know what is available, what are the risks and what are the benefits. My hope is that this information will be of use to you in making up your mind.

However, just in case you're still not comfortable with the idea, just in case you still think that you're not right for any of these procedures or believe that they're just for the rich and famous, I leave you with the results of the 2008 survey conducted by the American (Society of Aeatheic Plastic Surgeons (ASAPS). The 40-page document is a treasure trove of information:

♦ The most common surgical procedures: liposuction, eyelid jobs and nose jobs.

♦ The most common non-surgical procedures: Botox, microdermabrasion ("sanding" technique using a high speed rotating wheel to peel away skin), and chemical peels.

♦ Nose job season: Most nose jobs are done in the summer. Nose jobs have increased 46% since 1997.

♦ When most people tend to get plastic surgery: Winter.

♦ Why people travel 50 miles or more to get plastic surgery, if they have a qualified surgeon close to home: They want a vacation-like setting in which to recover.

♦ Percentage of plastic surgery patients who previously had plastic surgery: 30%.

♦ Percentage of plastic surgery patients who have had multiple procedures in the same year: 47%.

♦ Average cost of a Botox treatment (for one area) in 2008: 626

Perhaps the most fun is the "trends" page. It shows that:

♦ 36% of plastic surgeons saw a couple that underwent surgery together.

♦ 25% saw a mother and daughter who had surgery together.

♦ 31% saw a patient who received plastic surgery as a gift.

♦ 6% saw sisters having plastic surgery together.

♦ 4% saw friends having plastic surgery together.

What an excellent idea! When you do visit my office, please do bring a friend.

## The Future

Ponce de Leon failed in his search and gray hair and wrinkles remain part of life. Researchers will go on looking in other places for the scientific breakthrough that could preserve our youth and vitality forever—perhaps making all of these treatments obsolete.

As we age, the cells in our body are not able to grow and heal as quickly. Recently however, scientists have discovered how to outfox the body's slow deterioration (in one respect at least) by stimulating a gene called FoxM1B. By increasing the activity of the gene, researchers found that liver cells in old mice were able to grow as if the mice were still youngsters. And since the FoxM1B gene is found in many cells throughout the human body, some researchers believe this finding may one day be used to replace aging cells with young, new ones that could revitalize exhausted body organs.

Who knows what this discovery or others like it will bring? I and other good physicians are following it carefully and are at all times concerned with the health and happiness of you, our patients. We continue to search out and provide services that can enhance your appearance and self-esteem.

CPSIA information can be obtained at www.ICGtesting.com
Printed in the USA
LVOW10s0536031214

416526LV00002B/33/P

9 780986 520389